THE CANDY IN MY POCKET

THE WILD AND CRAZY LIFE OF A TYPE 1 DIABETIC

John Robert Wiltgen

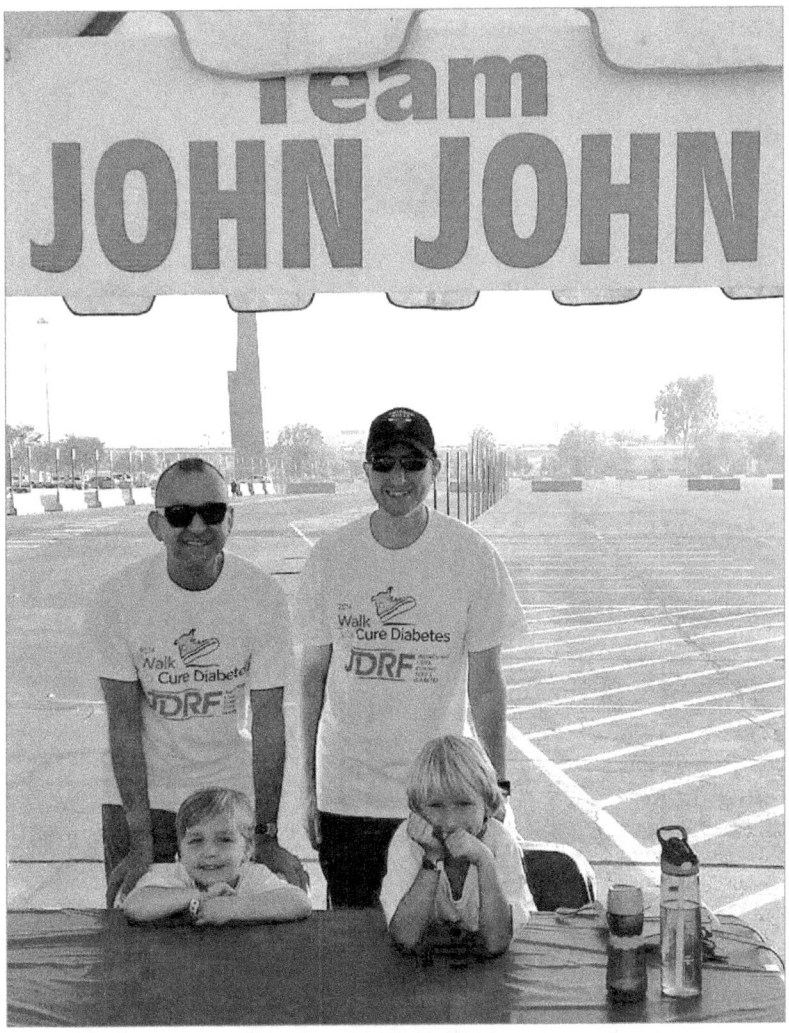

From left to right: John Robert Wiltgen with his nephew Justin, his brother-in-law John, and his nephew Travis, who walked in the Orange County walk-a-thon to help raise money for the Juvenile Diabetes Research Foundation.

A percentage of the profits from the sale of this book will be donated to the Juvenile Diabetes Research Foundation.

For media inquiries, questions about bulk purchases, permission to use any of the content of this book, or speaking availability, please visit www.thecandyinmypocket.com.

Library of Congress CIP is on file.

ISBNs:
979-8-9860070-0-7 (hardcover)
979-8-9860070-2-1 (paperback)
979-8-9860070-1-4 (ebook)

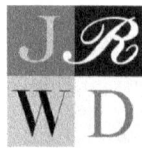

For my Mom, who I can never thank enough for putting up with all my crazy escapades and more importantly for giving me a second chance at life. I am sorry I gave you gray hair although it looks beautiful on you.

For my husband, Steven, who has also endured a lot of crazy adventures, never left my side, led prayer groups for me when my physicians thought I was going (and I don't mean First Class to San Tropez) and who has loved me unconditionally.

For AJ, Amy, Aunt Bea, Chris, Cindy, Cynthia, Daniela, Francine, Gera-Lind, Ivan, Jacqui, Jeff, Jill, Jimmy, Kiyoko, Lara, Leana, Leslie, Maxine, Mery, Miss Hollywood, Mr. Bill, Pat, Ray C, Ray W, Regina, Rhonda, Susan B, Susan H, Susan T, Willy and so many others. I am so thankful for our times together. My life would not have been the same without you.

For my clients. You believed in me and my visions for your residences. Your homes are beautiful because you let them be. Thank you.

Finally, for my doctors and your assistants. You know where I would be without you. Thank you for never giving up on me.

Table of Contents

INTRODUCTION ix

COO, COO, CA-CHOO, Mrs. ROBINSON 1

FRANKY AND JOHNNY 23

DIAGNOSIS DIABETES 39

CRAZY WORLD 44

A BETTER ME 49

THE ODD COUPLE 52

IN A NEW YORK MINUTE 56

DOCTOR MY EYES 68

DOWNTOWN 75

THAT'S WHERE THE HAPPY PEOPLE GO 83

A STAR IS BORN 91

THE SHOW MUST GO ON 94

HELP ME 103

CAN YOU SEE ME NOW? 109

WORKIN' DAY AND NIGHT 119

DO YOU WANT TO DANCE? 122

THE PARTY'S OVER 129

WHAT'S UP DOC? 135

RECYCLE KIDNEYS NOT JUST DIET COKE CANS 148

I CAN ONLY BE ME 153

THE HOUSE THAT BUILT ME 190

COUNT YOUR BLESSINGS 196

TWO AMERICANS IN PARIS 200

LIVIN' LA VIDA LOCA 209

NOBODY WALKS IN LA 212

FOREVER IS AS LONG AS IT LASTS 231

IT'S A JUNGLE OUT THERE 238

WE ARE FAMILY 250

SOMETHING ABOUT JANE SEYMOUR 253

WHO COULD ASK FOR ANYTHING MORE? 259

THE GERMAN POPE, THE WEDDING AND THE NOSE JOB 265

TAKE A LOAD OFF YOUR FEET 270

SOURAND SWEET 279

ME AND Mr. JONES 283

HIS EXCELLENCY 290

UNDER AFRICAN SKIES 295

AFRICAN REGGAE 310

MORE AFRICAN REGGAE 313

ISTANBUL NOT CONSTANTINOPLE 324

OUT OF AFRICA 332

RUNNING UP THAT HILL 337

IN CASE OF FIRE KEEP CALM AND PUT YOUR LEG ON 343

LIVING IN AMERICA 350

BABY YOU CAN DRIVE MY CAR 355

I LOOK TO YOU 359

I'M STILL HERE 369

INTRODUCTION

I knew I was destined for greatness when Zsa Zsa Gabor said I should be on stage. Yes, me! But then, I felt afraid there could be a black cloud in my future when Sid Caesar told me, "If you don't have tragedy, you won't have comedy. Crying and laughing are the same thing, but you can never laugh too hard."

My memoir is about just that: creating your best life possible and staying positive despite terrible circumstances. This book chronicles my dramatic days as a top designer commissioned by celebrities, world leaders, and other luminaries; my (secret) debilitating and death-defying battle with diabetes; and my struggle to hold on to myself and those I cared about along the way.

I wrote this to help people of all beliefs and backgrounds remain optimistic in the worst of times—no matter what personal or professional challenges you're dealing with. And my goal is to help raise awareness about the deadly but little-known symptoms and consequences of diabetes (a group of metabolic disorders characterized by high blood sugar levels over a prolonged period).

This debilitating disease at least doubles a person's risk of an early loss of life. As of 2019, it was the cause of approximately 4.2 million global deaths for the estimated 463 million people worldwide diagnosed with type 1 or type 2 diabetes. It can cause many serious long-term complications including amputation, blindness, cardiovascular disease, Charcot foot, cognitive impairment, gastroparesis, kidney failure, nerve damage, and stroke.

You might not have diabetes or know someone who does, but we all have challenges and need stories exemplifying how to live our best lives, or at least laugh while trying! This is not a self-help or "What to do" book. It's really a "What *not* to do" book. My memoir doesn't contain much medical information. I am not going to write about Joseph von Mering and Oskar Minkowski who discovered the role of the pancreas in diabetes back in 1889.

More than anything, it's a fun and adventurous, sometimes scary story that will take you out of your life, around the world, and then, leave you in a better place than when you started. At least that's my intent.

I was diagnosed with "juvenile" diabetes in 1967 and battled the complications throughout my adult life. With just three years of high school and less at design school, I managed to build an internationally recognized, award-winning design firm. The youngest designer to receive the Merchandise Mart's "Outstanding Achievement in the Design Profession" award, John Robert Wiltgen Design collected 44 other accolades. I have been responsible for everything from the Steve Harvey penthouse in Trump Tower Chicago to a 40,000 square foot estate on the island of Ikoyi, Lagos (Nigeria).

Many of the homes I've designed have been featured on HGTV and NBC's "Open House," or were published in 200+ newspaper and magazine stories. That said, this book is for *you*. It's a confirmation that any adversity you're dealing with is worth fighting. And a reminder that you're wiser than you and maybe those around you realize. You know what to do. We all do. We simply need "sweet reminders" along the way.

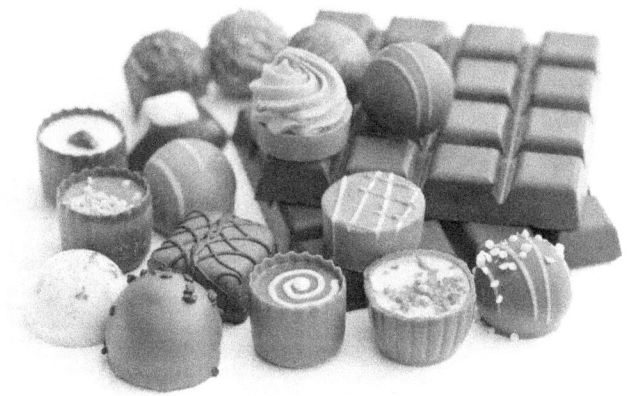

COO, COO, CA-CHOO, Mrs. ROBINSON

Paul stormed into the office screaming at Sharon as if she caused it all. My receptionist grabbed her female belly Russian lynx coat and bolted.

The next thing I knew, Paul and I were fighting. A real brawl. Something at which he was much better than I. Trying to escape the same way Sharon did, he caught up with me in the hallway, threw me down on the dirty bottle green and beige pindot carpeting and leaned over my powerless form with a hammer-like fist raised to attack.

Not knowing what else to do, I kicked him in the face with my Gucci riding boot, which I purchased before I bought my horse.

He was stunned, but that made him even angrier. Paul was poised to reshape my four-eyed face when the namesake of Francis J. Barbaria Interiors, Inc. emerged from his office across the hall and swiftly pointed a shiny silver handgun at Paul's head.

"I suggest you get off that young man," he commanded in the unruffled tone of someone who knew how to pull the trigger.

***

In September 1976, at the tender age of 17, I became the youngest branch manager in the history of the SCM Glidden Paint Corp. I hopped on its bandwagon while loitering in one of their stores close to my parent's home in Arlington Heights, eventually landing a paying job there. Later I was transferred to a different location and shortly thereafter named manager of the Midwest Region's model branch.

After three years, I had it with high school and therefore, didn't return for my senior year. Thanks to my extra classes and independent studies in art, theatre and business I accumulated enough credits to graduate. With Leana (the love of my life) off to ASU in the fall on an art scholarship, I couldn't fathom being there without her. The promotion to Glidden's newest store came at the perfect time.

I felt I made the big time with my private almond-colored office with an executive desk and leather swivel chair. In it I hung this gigantic painting of the Grand Canyon I created in art class with a palette knife and acrylic paints. My position came with a young secretary. Well, not that young. She was older than me. To be honest, everyone was older than me, including my 54-year-old assistant manager.

Whoever said, "timing is everything," knew exactly what they were talking about.

As a provision of the promotion elevating me to a higher ego bracket, I had to promise not to tell anyone how old I wasn't.

My boss worried that tenured employees would march out the corporate door if they learned how quickly I sprinted up the Glidden ladder. Of course, I agreed without even knowing what "tenured" meant.

Although the position, given my age, was unbelievable, it did little to advance my artistic career. The more I thought about Leana, the more I longed to be doing something creative too.

Leana. She's Macedonian, meaning she comes from the same place as Alexander the Great. She is short. Back then she had long dark hair. Huge, hypnotizing, dark brown eyes and beautiful olive colored skin. In high school she was a size 13, because—as she professed—she had big bones. Although later in life she became an eight. (Her bones must have shrunk.) And she was a 36C.

That never changed.

She was a dancer in Orchesis and an upper classman. I was a sophomore when we met; she a junior. I showed her the big city like no one else could and she showed me a thing or two.

Well, one thing for sure. I was raised believing you weren't supposed to do *that* until you were married but she convinced me otherwise.

We were attached at the hip for years and fought like an old married couple because both of us were always right. I thought about her studying art in a far-away college. I had no idea where Tempe, Arizona was except you had to fly to Phoenix to get there.

She won a full four-year scholarship. It was the only way she could go to college as her parents refused to support her. There were no congratulatory words of encouragement. They did not send her money for food, books or art supplies. Their beliefs included higher education was for men, but Leana's place was in their home until she married anyone but me.

Working at Sadie Thompson's, a Phoenix restaurant providing food, booze and boogie, she was too young to serve liquor, so Leana was a dime-a-dance girl. Orchesis and all our disco dancing paid off.

I wrote her almost every day. She responded often, drawing skillfully on the outside of her envelopes with colored pencils, crayons, and spray paint. Each one was an original work of art filled with so many emotions, so much love. I should have saved them. She inspired me to change my life.

When I found out what my managerial benefits package included, I enrolled in night classes at Ray Vogue School of Design while managing the paint store by day. It was located downtown on Chicago's famed Magnificent Mile (Michigan Avenue north of the river). The school offered programs in professional art, photography, fashion and interior design. The thought of it made me oyfgehaytert and I'm not even Jewish.

Although art classes did not seem the ideal choice for a corporate manager, Glidden paid for it. And so did Dad. He had no idea about my company subsidies, and I didn't tell him, so I made money going to school.

The Ray Vogue classroom is where I first laid eyes on HER. Not yet 18, my life embraced some mega turns dragging me, all too willingly, into adulthood. The most gorgeous female I ever encountered was in my class. Dazzling red hair, a peaches and cream complexion, and fashionably dressed. Her shoes and handbags were not just shoes and handbags, they were stylishly sculpted works of art. In high school Leana worked part-time at Carol Casuals, but she sold nothing remotely close to what this gorgeous Aphrodite-like goddess wore. Always perfectly put together. She had to be a size 2 with the most beautiful smile and distinguished laugh. The problem was, she sat on the other side of the room.

I had to get closer.

Trying to be inconspicuous, each week I moved to a chair closer to hers. Our seats were not assigned although that wouldn't have stopped me. While I had not yet learned her name, she was my reason for not cutting class—a maneuver I mastered in high school. Her aura inspired me to be more creative while learning everything I could. She motivated me to ace my assignments. My muse.

After months of lessons, our instructor gave us floor plans to design, render and present to him in front of our fellow classmates. Mine was a master bedroom which I hoped to create rivaling those in glossy magazines.

Starting with a lavish tented bed centered in the room it was complimented with a hand carved antique armoire to conceal a television (they were boxy and heavy in those days). A pair of armless upholstered chairs in the window were placed around an occasional table and acrylic lamp. Multicolored striped silk draperies were lined with a bright, sunny solid. In the center of all that a geometric patterned comforter.

Dennis, our instructor, had a considerable lisp. I never heard anyone speak like that except Zsa Zsa Gabor's hairdresser, Pierre, who repeatedly told me I was a nice boy which freaked me out. After listening to my presentation, I expected Dennis to order me to start over. But with one glance, in front of the entire class, he said "Sfabulous."

I was so proud, even more proud after class. While packing my portfolio, Rhonda—yes, finally, that was her name— approached me, saying how much she loved my bedroom. If she only knew what my bedroom in the moldy basement of my parents' modest suburban home looked like.

At the next class I sat right next to her.

She and I became fast friends while cutting fabric swatches for our presentation boards or working on floorplans and renderings of rooms we were designing. She'd ask me for my opinion. In return, I'd do the same. Loving the camaraderie in class, I was miserable when the two hours were finished Tuesday and Thursday nights.

Wanting to impress Rhonda, I boasted of my managerial position with Glidden Paint where we sold paint. And wallpaper! And I told her about Leana and her art scholarship at ASU.

In return, Rhonda told me she was already designing people's homes. She had her own business which made me the one who was impressed.

After class, we would stop at the diner on the school's first floor. Charmette's. Rhonda ordered an exotic beverage called Espresso. To my disappointment, it was a little cup of strong coffee. I ordered Tab to wash down my chocolate sundae as there was no such thing as Diet Coke yet.

Ice cream was a stupid choice. Was I still rebelling against the restrictive nature of my diabetes management? I felt fine. That's what mattered. Others enjoyed desserts, why not me? It wasn't denial. It was medical oblivion. I had a sweet tooth and no real clue yet about diabetic complications.

One balmy evening Rhonda and I lingered after class. In a conversation lasting longer than I realized, she pointed to the gold watch peeking from an array of bracelets dangling from her wrist, reminding me it was time to catch my train.

"No. I was running late at work, so I drove in today," I replied. "Can I give you a lift?"

"I live just a few blocks away. I can walk." After months of schooling together I still knew very little about her.

"If it's only a few blocks, then it will only take a few minutes. It would be my pleasure," I was persistent.

After several more rounds of "no, it's really not necessary" and "please, it's no inconvenience," she agreed.

"Great. My car is in the garage half a block down the street."

Approaching 11 pm, the city streets were filled with people enjoying the weather. An attendant delivered my 1964 Cadillac Sedan de Ville. The Matador Red factory paint job with white leather interior and white rag top accentuated the long, sleek shape of the body with fins. It was 14 years old, but a showpiece. All heads turned when I barreled down the highway and I was VERY proud of my first car. Bought it before I even had a driver's license. So glad I had it washed earlier in the day. Rhonda looked surprised as the car-hiker held the door open for her.

"Is *this* your car?"

Trying to appear the debonair sophisticate, I shot a smile showing off teeth my parents' numerous financial sacrifices braced. Giggling, she climbed in, telling me to turn left onto Michigan Avenue towards Water Tower Place the city's glamorous vertical shopping mall that included boutiques such as

Yves St. Laurent, Halston and Fiorucci. That's where the Ritz-Carlton Hotel is hidden too.

"Okay. Turn right," directed Rhonda, and a few seconds later, "Okay. Stop." In all, the ride was two and a half blocks.

I gazed at the all too familiar home of my former study hall (when I cut class in high school). "I don't get it. This is the Ritz…"

"This is where I live," she said, batting her mesmerizing lashes in my direction.

"You live here?" I gulped.

She flipped her flowing red mane over a shoulder and said "Yes. This is where I live. Do you want to come up?"

Oh my God. The most expensive condominium development in Chicago, at that time, was the one above the Ritz Carlton Hotel. Until that night she had been the bait, but her Water Tower condo hooked me.

"Uhm. Sure. What should I do with my car?"

"Just leave it here. I'll tell the doormen you are coming up for a little while."

She whispered something to one of the uniformed men watching me maneuver my car as coolly as I could. He nodded.

The guarded doors to the private residences are just east of the hotel entrance. The attendants smiled and greeted us. "Good evening, sir. Good evening Mrs. Byron."

BADA BOOM! That was my heart sinking through the marble floor.

She's married! How old is she?

A yappy long-haired Dachshund named Kelly greeted us at the door of her 42nd floor home. I wasn't sure what to expect. Would there be a yappy husband too?

Nope.

The coast was clear. After explaining they were separated, she invited me in. The foyer floor was covered with large ceramic tiles emblazoned with green and yellow flowers.

Interesting.

A large white sofa sat on a lime green shag rug in front of the living room windows featuring a breathtaking view overlooking East Lake Shore Drive, the beach, and lake. I couldn't believe she invited me in to visit her world.

Her master bedroom featured a bottle green suede upholstered bed surrounded by L-shaped ottomans hugging the corners. It was exquisite. The matching suede coverlet was accented with white fur pillows.

Why was she in school?

When the tour ended, she asked me to sit in the living room with her, but I had to leave. It was past midnight and a 45-minute drive home. I was opening the store at 7 am. That called for another 45-minute drive after shaving, showering, dressing and taking my shot (of insulin).

After that night, we were inseparable, though I remained faithful to Leana. Rhonda didn't have to twist my arm to accompany her to parties. The rooftops of buildings in Streeterville. A Lake Shore Drive condo. The Pump Room. Zorine's, a private supper club/disco with its dancing waiters and acrylic staircases. Most of the guests at these places were twice my age. Old enough to be my parents. Maybe older. But my accomplishments entitled me to be there too as I secretly wondered: why was I living and working in the suburbs? I belonged in the city. But, because I was only 17, I couldn't yet sign a lease to rent my own apartment.

It didn't take long for me to follow Rhonda's example and start a side business bearing my name. My teacher, Dennis, suggested a predominantly black fold over business card with white ink. Said it would make a great first impression and first impressions are lasting ones.

I saved the names of good customers from the paint stores who, I suspected, could afford the services of an aspiring and EXTREMELY young interior designer. Later, I would design entire houses from the ground up, pools, even gardens and my cards would read… "architectural, interior and landscape design", but back then, I sent a lot of letters with some photographs of renderings (school projects), hoping to attract a client or two who were interested in some creative furniture plans and gorgeous designer furnishings.

Those efforts brought me my first commission. A doctor's wife responded. She and her husband lived near the hospital in Arlington Heights (my hometown) and needed help furnishing their residence. Rhonda also recommended me to a suburban couple with whom she didn't want to work because of the commute.

"But do not let them know how young you are," she cautioned.

***

In January 1978, returning from a very steamy (sometimes clumsy) 10-day winter vacation with Leana in Arizona, I tendered my two weeks' notice at the paint store. I decided to go back to school full time, also taking evening and Saturday classes. That schedule would enable me to earn my degree in half the time.

The regional manager for Glidden, my immediate boss, was shocked. I had been manager for 16 months and he expected me to be there forever, at least until the SCM Glidden Corp had a chance to give me a gold watch. (I'd already been to one of those corporate functions, which was another reason I wanted out.) He pleaded with me to stay longer. My assistant manager had no idea how to reconcile inventory or follow up on payment requisitions to vendors. But my mind was made up. I was certain Glidden could find a tenured employee to fill my shoes.

I packed my office and tied the Grand Canyon painting to the roof of my car. Jerry, my outside sales rep, helped. As everyone bade farewell it was exhilarating to know I was getting the hell out of Dodge to make a new life in the Windy City.

Zooming down the tollway at a speed greater than that posted on the roadside signs, the wind caught my four-by-six-foot painting, tore the ropes holding it down and lifted it off the roof of my car. In the rear-view mirror, I could see it fly over cars behind me, but… I just kept going. There was no turning back.

On Tuesday and Thursday nights I saw Rhonda. After class, we changed into runway-looking attire and headed for *Faces*, a private disco with its sci-fi-like mirrored tunnel leading to the glamorous interior where we danced the night away. Her best friend AJ often accompanied us. We were like the three musketeers marching up and down Rush Street. Many times we were out all night, so if I remembered to bring insulin and a syringe, I stayed overnight at Rhonda's. If not, at 4:00 in the morning I drove her husband's Monte Carlo home, which was conveniently parked in the Water Tower Place garage. Bobby Womack's "*Daylight*" became my theme song…

…and it looks like daylight is going to catch me up again.

Most people are getting up when I'm just getting in…

School came in handy. I was designing several homes, so I used classroom time to develop those projects. I earned money and credit for my work at the same time. One morning, in the middle of a lecture, I got up, grabbed my coat and excused myself. The teacher told me to sit down. I told her of my meeting with a client at the Mart and had to leave.

That didn't impress her.

She said I was insubordinate and told me to take my seat. I left anyway. I wasn't going to let her tell me what to do. When I returned after a very profitable meeting and delicious lunch, there was a note taped to my locker. The headmaster summoned me.

The meeting was brief. He was pleasant while instructing me to clean out my industrial gray colored locker. There was no need to pay the next installment of my tuition. After four months as a full-time student, I was dismissed from Ray Vogue School of Design.

Forever.

Why did I quit my job at Glidden? I went home to meditate before meditating was a thing.

I wasn't used to being told what to do. On the contrary, I told my employees in the store what to do. That's the way I liked it. I'm German and a Leo.

After some research, I was offered a job at Petersen Interiors, a high-end contemporary furniture studio, exactly one block from Arlington Heights High School where I was a student two years ago. With my qualifications, the store manager wanted me to start immediately. The problem was, I didn't want to work there and desperately looked for other options.

I needed to escape the suburbs.

Rhonda suggested another opportunity. Friends of hers owned a furniture manufacturer with a 6,000 square foot Merchandise Mart showroom needing a manager. I was born to be a manager and longed to be downtown. In the Mart was even better. It was like a city unto itself. It even had its own zip code. I took that job.

Berne Furniture manufactured upholstered pieces in Berne, Indiana. Amish factory workers crafted the most beautiful solid hardwood frames with double doweled corner blocks and hand tied hour-glass coil springs that came with a life-time guarantee. Unfortunately, they were upholstered in God awful covers and marketed mostly through very rural retail stores. For the showroom, I was instructed to "jazz" it up a bit and order semi-truckloads of their furniture in urban appropriate fabrics.

I loved the challenge.

On weekends I would push and pull different pieces of furniture around the showroom to make the groupings more interesting. The best groupings I placed near the entry so everyone that walked by could see them.

Berne's owners were undertakers who also made coffins like so many furniture companies. They owned two funeral homes, one in Berne, the other on Paradise Island, Bahamas.

After having settled into my new position, the FBI came to the showroom—not to buy a sofa sectional. Showing me their badges, which looked authentic, they started asking questions about the Paradise Island funeral parlor. Had I been there? Did I know anything about its manager?

No. All I knew about the Bahamas, I told them, was my dad went there once with some girlfriend which made Mom terribly angry and depressed.

It was the truth.

Several months later Rhonda told me the Bahamian manager was found guilty of stuffing drugs into the cavities of dead bodies before shipping them to the US. In those coffins made in Berne, Indiana by Mennonites.

While managing the showroom, Rhonda would stop by to hang up her coat before shopping for her clients. When she was done for the day, we would go through her bag of tricks. Fabrics. Wallpaper samples. Photos of furniture she was liking for a project. The goddess always asked for my opinion batting her long eyelashes at me.

One day she dropped a bomb. A HUGE ONE. Rhonda proposed we start a design firm together—the two of us. Living in the most expensive condominium tower in Chicago and divorcing a very accomplished man, she wanted ME to be her business partner.

Before long, Byron, Wiltgen and Associates, Inc. became a full-time business with a handful of part-time employees. Rhonda was, as it turned out, also a United Airlines flight attendant (something I didn't know until we discussed me quitting my Berne Furniture job). However, she had seniority and promised to work the minimum number of trips so she could work the maximum number of hours by my side. We rented a small office in a building immediately behind the Mart.

It had two big windows and a panoramic view of the El tracks. Each time a train passed, which was often, we had to put our phone calls on hold.

Great beginnings!

Rhonda and I were equal partners and owning our own business came with great benefits. The company even bought us a corporate membership to Huckleberry's (Barbara Eden's private supper club / disco on Oak Street). It had a glass elevator connecting the dining room to the dance club and was the hottest place for several years. We entertained clients there or at Zorine's, ultimately ending up at Faces, which was always filled with traders, sports figures, models and movie stars. To me, it was the big time. I wasn't even old enough to drink, although, thanks to fake ID's, I had been for years.

Who'd have thought I'd not only be running around town with the most striking creature on the planet, but she'd also be my business partner?

While dining at the Pump Room one evening, she suggested we sell her soon-to-be-ex-husband Paul 10 percent of our respective 50 percent ownerships. This would provide him an incentive to do our books inexpensively (he was the comptroller for a big-time pharmaceutical company) and refer clients to us through his professional and social connections. We needed that. I agreed. At 18, and with my very limited education, it sounded like a smart play, so Rhonda and I each ended up owning 40 percent of our design firm and Paul 20 percent.

Our first job for a developer, was to design a model home in Chicago's Gold Coast. Our friend Shayle was renovating a vintage rental apartment building into pricey condominiums lacking amenities and parking. But they were large with high ceilings, lots of chunky moldings, wood burning fireplaces in the living and primary bedrooms and no views.

Having spent so much time in Rhonda's Water Tower Place condo, it was hard to imagine why someone might choose to live in a building with no doormen or health club. But imagine we did. Once the furniture and artwork selections were delivered and installed, we were hired by people who bought in the building and others who viewed our work.

Shayle remains my friend to this very day. He is proud of the fact he commissioned us to design our very first model home. Telling everyone he launched my career; I remind him he only hired us because he was anxious to climb into Rhonda's bed. With her in it, of course.

Unlike my parents who were divorced several years before, Paul and Rhonda remained friendly, which shocked me. I thought divorced people were supposed to hate one another. But the three of us and sometimes others would go out for dinner. Together. Four and five courses while this was going on.

When the divorce was final, I organized a "Congratulations on Your Divorce" party for her which featured a cake broadcasting it in butter cream frosting. Unexpectedly, Paul walked into our office decorated with balloons and saw us drinking champagne and eating cake. He stormed out like a kid who just had his pants pulled down and spanked.

Paul kept the Water Tower Place condo. Rhonda received cash and a parcel of land on California's coast near Bodega where Alfred Hitchcock filmed *The Birds*. They got joint custody of the dog. She bought a condo in a more modest high-rise and suggested I also buy one in the same building.

"Sure. Why not?"

I was under her spell and would do anything she told me to. Anything. Was that because I found out Leana was having an affair with her "life" drawing teacher? I don't think so. Being so far away from one another, we grew apart. I had a new life downtown. And, she obviously had a new one too.

Sayonara baby!

After signing the papers for the purchase of my condo, I went home for dinner. Bad Daddy was there too.

"Guess what I bought today?"

Mom, "A new suit?"

"No."

Dad, "A new car?"

"No. I bought a condo."

"You bought what?" he was shocked. Then, jealously, "They won't let you buy a condo. YOU'RE TOO YOUNG."

Well, obviously, he didn't know the same "They" I knew. My "They" were fine with my age.

"Hmmmph," was his boneheaded comment before, "I suppose Mrs. Robinson put you up to this?"

That was how Mom referred to Rhonda. Now my father, too. I could understand Mom's synonym for her, but Dad's infidelities made him the "Mr. Robinson." Who was he to judge me?

What would we do without culturally significant films to educate us about the real world?

***

After an extremely busy October, Rhonda and I needed a night out. It was Halloween. First a costume party at the apartment of our friends Sue and Cynthia who I knew through Leana. Sue used to be in an art class with her at ASU and Cynthia was one of Leana's roommates. She suggested Cynthia, who always sewed her own clothes, switch from fine art to fashion design. Taking her advice, Cynthia moved back to Chicago and enrolled at the Art Institute.

Rhonda and I dressed as mimes, wearing Cappezio tight, black, lycra body stockings with white collars and cuffs. The costume embarrassed me as it showed off all my… assets. But Rhonda said we looked great, and I would never argue with her.

After dancing the conga with 50 other costumed guests down the street, into the Emerald Isle Pub, around and back to the party house, we were ready to dance on. Better music. So Rhonda and I hopped in a cab and went to Coconuts (yet another supper club/disco, although this one was not for members' only). She desperately wanted to hear Blondie's *Heart of Glass* and after many spins around the dance floor it was finally time to go home.

We were in the cab. It was 3 am. I glanced at her. She looked at me. It was not like any of the other times. Our eyes locked. For the first time, I kissed her on the mouth. Hard. She kissed me back. Neither of us cared about being in the back seat of a taxi. Our mouths and hands were all over each other.

At her home, Rhonda poured herself a glass of wine and opened a can of Tab for me, then disappeared. I heard the tub filling. She reappeared wearing something too sheer to be a bath robe. She told me to remove my smelly body stocking and get into the tub.

What to do?

I wasn't sure, but it did not take a second request. The tub was surrounded with lit candles. Rhonda climbed in on top of me. We hastily began exploring each other in the steamy confines of the small tub. I was young and hard but had an intense case of blue balls and came quickly. After drying each other off, we slipped between the silk sheets of her king size bed. It provided much more room for us to discover each other and in the most unusual positions. She was much more creative than I as she pushed my head between her legs.

There were many nights like that …

We were enjoying our newfound intimacy when the phone rang. It was the doorman. At 5:00 in the morning. Ray was in the lobby with a young lady and wanted to come up. My 16-year-old brother and his girlfriend were at the same costume party. They were a little over served (self-served is more like it) and on their way home when he made a wrong turn getting on the expressway. They ended up on the south side of Chicago (the totally opposite direction of our home in the northwest suburbs) where he got a flat tire. And no spare. Wearing nothing but a grass skirt and combat boots with his girlfriend in a very authentic looking fringed flapper dress, they stood on the shoulder of the expressway and hitched a ride back into the city.

***

There was a lot going on at home I knew very little about. Sometime after Mom divorced my father (a mortal sin) they started dating each other. My father made nice, so she welcomed his sweetness and fawning. Was it because she was afraid of being alone? Or overwhelmed about where a divorced woman with four kids might find another man? He was a good bullshitter and five years after divorcing Bad Daddy she remarried him in St. James Catholic church. With their newer guitar accompanied sermons it was more progressive than the church we attended for years. Now, Mom didn't have to worry about God, whom she loved and feared at the same time. But His church was no longer the problem. Remarrying my father was.

***

Byron, Wiltgen and Associates continued to grow. We were designing a variety of prestigious projects. Corporate head-quarters. Luxurious private residences throughout the city and suburbs. Model homes scattered about the Chicagoland area—our best advertising. Rhonda and I acted as designers, financial planners, contract negotiators, general contractors, even publicists. Other flight attendants who married well heard about us through Rhonda and AJ as they all flew the friendly skies. I began to dream big. Unfortunately, I didn't realize that golden times tend to make the gods jealous.

In less than 18 months, our brand gained a reputation for transforming spaces with outstanding results. But increasingly Rhonda was spending less time working while still collecting her salary. And less time with me. Was I just imagining it? It took me some time to decide.

I was heart-broken to learn she was jet-setting with a direc-tor of Playboy Enterprises. Rhonda and I kept our personal relationship private, so no one in our office knew anything about the two of us. Our secretary, Sharon, also a United

Airlines flight attendant, unknowingly spilled the beans. Rhonda had been "seeing" this high-powered executive for a while.

People love to gossip.

When I confronted Rhonda, she defensively explained she visited some Playboy resorts, hoping to convince their management team that our firm should design their properties. Unbelievable. That was something I hadn't even dreamt of, probably because I never stayed in a resort.

I wanted to believe her.

When Sharon's ugly rumors proved not to be rumors, I visited Paul in his Water Tower bachelor pad to ask his advice. Afterall, he owned 20% of us so this affected him too. I only discussed the business side of the situation. I knew enough to not discuss anything about our personal relationship. Despite the divorce, Paul remained very protective of Rhonda. I would soon learn just how protective. He was 50 and the size of a football linebacker. I was 19 and shaped like a string bean. And if you took the average of our two ages, Mrs. Robinson was 35. A long time elapsed before I learned that about her.

Still wet from his shower, Paul greeted me wearing a towel and holding the long-haired dachshund. Kelly kept yapping at window washers spritzing and squeegeeing the 42nd floor windows. While I had much to discuss, it was impossible— the dog continued to distract everyone. Paul walked over to the window giving Kelly a better view of the workmen. In the commotion, Paul's towel dropped to the floor.

Fortunately, the window washers were harnessed to a mechanical lift.

I never learned why the laborers laughed so hard. Paul dropped the dog to pick up his towel covering himself before turning around and sitting at the glass dining table. We discussed Rhonda and her absence from the office. I professed I was working twice as hard to keep up with our work demands and felt we should either reduce her pay or increase mine. After a lengthy discussion (I did most of the talking), he nodded and said he would speak with her. A situation solved, I thought, proud of my sure-footed diplomacy.

The next day Sharon said Paul was on line 1 and didn't sound happy. I immediately picked up the phone. He accused me of having an affair with his wife. I assured him nothing happened while they were married. I said our personal relationship, following their divorce, was totally unexpected and short lived, so it now seemed.

The phone went dead.

Twenty minutes later, Paul flew into the office in a rage. Before long, we were fighting. Just like in some John Wayne movie. Only there weren't any bar stools. Probably because we were in the hallway of our office building. But before he knew it Paul found himself looking directly into the muzzle of Frank's gun. Shocked, he picked himself up and sprinted to the elevators.

FRANKY
AND JOHNNY

Frank, short for Francis, led me into his office to calm me down. My Byron, Wiltgen and Associates office across the hall was strictly utilitarian (a clever use of a limited amount of space) while Frank's was gracious and almost, well, aristocratic. Exquisite period furniture. Original artwork. Pre-Columbian antiquities. This man was a very well-seasoned professional designer. Despite my accomplishments, I felt sophomoric by comparison. His secretary, Jerry, brought me a Tab in a gleaming cut crystal glass. We began the office tour accompanied by Leoncavallo's *Pagliacci*, an opera featuring a clown who is happy on the outside, but miserable inside. Only Frank and Jerry occupied the striking five-room studio.

He resembled an Italian movie star from a neo-realist Roberto Rossellini film. Glossy, thick, dark wavy hair. Matching full bushy eyebrows. Clear green eyes. He was abbronzatura and impeccably dressed.

Invigorated by the recent fiasco, he wanted a full briefing on Paul. Why was he about to beat the shit out of me? Frank was eager to learn everything. I explained how Rhonda and I met, became business partners and had a short, now-cooled personal relationship. He asked my age.

Everyone wanted to know that.

Not yet 20, he marveled I had an older business partner/lover and surmised I must have… many talents. He let me ramble for quite some time. Then he surreptitiously checked his gleaming gold Piaget watch.

"Oh, I'm sorry," I apologized. "I didn't mean to take up so much of your time. You've been very kind and I'm sure you have better things to do."

"Nonsense," he replied theatrically. "The night is just beginning, but with all that excitement, I'm hungry. Aren't you?"

I cautiously nodded my head in agreement.

"Perfect. Let's go."

Rising dramatically from his seat, it was almost as if he was being levitated. He ran to his private office and returned bundled in a huge fur coat. Tanuki—a magical Japanese foxlike dog somewhat resembling raccoon. Once considered evil, Tanuki became an icon of generosity, cheer, and prosperity.

Who doesn't need plenty of that?

I had to go across the hall to retrieve my ivory wool sailor's pea coat, which I thought was "all that" until I got a glimpse of Frank's coat which was "all that" and more.

Frank accompanied me.

Though totally embarrassed by our limited space, my fear was Paul might return. With my knight in shining armor by my side, I nervously entered. The place was empty. No Paul. No Rhonda. And no Sharon.

Our long narrow space was divided into three sections: a reception/waiting area, an office Paul shared with a draftsman and a bunch of catalogs, and the studio with two tall windows facing the El tracks which Rhonda and I shared.

We left in a hurry.

At The Ritz, Frank was interested in my business. I was curious about Francis J. Barbaria Interiors. I described our 18 months' worth of design projects, told him about my managerial position with Glidden Paint, my work in the theatre—even my job being the best fish breader at Eddie's Lounge. He seemed genuinely impressed.

Well, maybe not about the fish.

In turn, he told me about himself. He was 40 (older than Mrs. Robinson), studied design at the Art Institute of Chicago, and visited his relatives in Sicily. Some of his considerable knowledge of art, furniture and design was acquired on his trips there. He also went on an archeological dig somewhere in the "boot," which helped refine his expertise in antiquities.

I was fascinated.

He mentioned some of his clients whose names meant nothing to me, but I understood they were the crème de la crème of Chicago society.

After dinner, Frank said he was having such a good time, he didn't want the evening to end. What else could we do? I was pleasantly surprised. It was nice to be interesting to someone, after almost being beaten up by Paul and deserted by Rhonda. I volunteered to show Frank an in-town, two-bedroom condominium we recently finished for clients who lived in Arizona.

"Yep, let's go," he agreed.

We parked his Mercedes in Lincoln Park and walked to 2800 Lake Shore Drive. The autumn air was brisk, particularly if you were the one not wearing the fur coat.

With the building's modern architecture in mind Rhonda and I designed this home to reflect the latest styling. Except for the textured ceramic tile in the entry and kitchen, we selected gray wall-to-wall plush carpeting for the rest of the interior. (This is in the '70's.) The furniture was a combination of lacquered linen, acrylic, leather, goatskin, and wood. The guest bedroom furniture was gloss Formica, a material taking the furniture industry by storm. Bleached wood nightstands, a lacquered dresser, and patent leather headboard completed the master bedroom.

Returning to the living room, we stood at the window savoring the striking view. I wondered what the "pro" truly thought of our installation. I was happy to have someone to share it with.

Standing there for a moment, Frank then turned, grabbed and kissed me. I was stunned. I'd never been kissed by a man. Not on the mouth. Not even when my junior high school friends and I played spin the bottle. Girls could kiss girls, but boys did not kiss boys. If the bottle pointed to another guy, we just spun it again.

I stopped kissing Dad when I was 6 or 7.

Frank kissed me again. Longer. Harder. Maybe there was some tongue. I was traumatized. When he let go, I jumped back.

"What?" he asked with a devilish smile.

I stuttered. "I have never done that before."

"What, kissed a man?"

"Yes."

"It's just like kissing a woman," he remarked like it was nothing unusual. "I live three blocks away. Do you want to see my place before you go home?"

Slowly I nodded my head.

"Where is home anyway?" he inquired.

"Well, it used to be in Old Town…" I started.

"You mean with Mrs. Byron?"

"Yes. No. I mean yes, well sort of," I wasn't sure what I meant. "When she left Water Tower Place, we each bought a condominium in a building on Wells Street. Then, when our relationship became personal I rented my place and stayed with her. Her place was bigger than my studio. Recently our affair ended, and I moved back to the suburbs at my family's home until my tenant's lease is up."

He ushered me out of my client's home, steered me towards the elevator, and when it opened, pushed me in and started kissing me again. He was a kissing maniac.

I should go straight home, I thought (like for a second).

But I was intrigued and wondered… what might happen next?

He wasn't lying about living three blocks away. His condo was in a 15-story neo-classic vintage midrise. The exterior was reminiscent of an old-world estate. We walked through a two-story arch in a thick limestone wall leading to a handsome courtyard. Despite my trepidations, I couldn't wait to see Frank's home.

When we exited the elevator, I was surprised. There were only two residences per floor. That possibility never dawned on me. The intimate reception area featured a stunning Biedermeier console with restrained geometric detailing. All I could think of was open the fucking door already. I wanted to see his home.

And I had to pee.

He must have heard me gasp. His place reflected my personal favorite style—Egyptian Revival. Since my childhood I dreamt of pyramids and sphinxes and the Mummy. I wanted to go to Cairo. Sail the Nile. Visit the Temples at Abu Simbel, Valley of the Kings, and Luxor. I'm convinced I lived there in a past life.

Frank's opulent setting included a colorful Egyptian border stenciled beneath the crown moldings. Three gilt bronze chandeliers, each with winged lionesses holding electrified candles romantically illuminated the space. A hand carved settee with animal legs and two reproduction throne chairs reminded me of the Treasures of Tutankhamen exhibit at the Chicago Art Institute.

When I was 16, I took Mom to see it for her 40th birthday celebration. Afterward we went to the Pump Room for lunch—to see and be seen. My treat. She loved it.

Frank's dining room was painted with larger-than-life images of assorted Egyptian gods. Ra, the God of the Sun. Osiris, the Lord of the Underworld. Isis, the Goddess of Magic and clever and ambitious women. She tricked Ra into retiring by poisoning him with a magic snake!

That whore! I'm surprised Ra did not have a magic snake of his own.

The bedroom walls were covered in delicate ivory linen on a gold metallic background. A sleigh bed upholstered in supple ivory leather was framed by ivory velvet draperies and a gold-fringed black velvet valance. The matching comforter was tactfully pulled back to reveal luxurious Italian linen sheets.

I wanted to live like this. And at various times in my life, I did. Starting that very night. Another awkward first for me. Very awkward. But where do you learn about these situations?

When I phoned Mom to check in the next morning, she told me Mrs. Robinson phoned. The goddess dropped another bomb. Not like the "let's be partners" bomb which was a good one. This one was the "you're fired" bomb similar to an atom bomb.

She and Paul decided I was no longer needed. Their decision was "effective immediately". No severance, whatever that was, and I had to give up my membership privileges to Huckleberry's.

Did she know when she suggested we sell Paul 20% of our company, the two of them would have 60% controlling interest? Did they scheme to use that to their benefit one day?

"You cannot be without insurance John. Make sure you track down your health insurance statement to determine it is paid and up to date." Those were Mom's parting words. She drilled that into my head when I turned 18, handing me my insurance bill guaranteeing me acceptance from our family's policy. I could never allow it to lapse. EVER. Because type 1 diabetes made me uninsurable.

I needed to drive to the suburbs for my morning shot of insulin. It was several hours past my scheduled dose, so I needed extra Regular to lower my blood glucose, which was sky high from all the craziness. Frank drove. He was especially attentive.

How did my life change so quickly? What did I do to bring out the Black Mambas in my partners? I worshipped Rhonda.

And respected her former husband. That black cloud Sid Caesar tried to prepare me for became a monsoon.

Frank hired me "effective immediately". I couldn't say no; he'd been too nice. Less than 24-hours after the Paul incident, my new boss dictated the first order of business. We were seeing a lawyer to file a lawsuit against Paul for assault and battery.

Blasting past the receptionists of the respected law firm Rooks, Pitts, Fullager and Poust, Frank was on a mission. Like a Tasmanian Devil, there was no stopping him. We proceeded to the office of his best friend and attorney, Terry Kiwala. The sudden intrusion did not faze Terry in the least. Frank ranted on and on about how Terry must file a lawsuit against Paul Byron for assaulting me. The settlement? Paul's Water Tower condo. While the idea of aggravating the Byron's was absolute nirvana for Frank, I wasn't sure. Neither was Terry.

A few days later Frank said, "We need a break. You've exhausted me." The next day we boarded a plane to Acapulco.

I'd been to Nogales, a Mexican border town, when I was a kid. Six months after I was diagnosed with diabetes my entire family went to Tucson on holiday. I think they too were exhausted.

As a diabetic I am a hand full and have exhausted a lot of people. Never on purpose.

Tucson was our home base. Mom used an 8mm camera to film a bunch of blue sky. No clouds. Sand. And Saguaro cactus. Dad drove us all over southern Arizona and to Mexico. We were there long enough to get some cheap souvenirs. Two natives whistled in harmony at my blonde haired, 7-year-old sister, which scared the living daylights out of Mother. She was afraid someone might kidnap Cindy. So we left. That's all I knew about the country south of the border.

***

I absolutely loved Acapulco.

Frank and I stayed right at a muggy hotel in the middle of the deep semicircular bay. The air conditioning didn't work. Thank God our room didn't get direct sun. The property was surrounded by lush flowering vegetation, tall palm trees and all sorts of lizards. Big ones. Little Ones.

Poisonous ones.

Frank would sleep in, but I was thrilled to walk the beach every morning. In the middle of the night the city tilled the fine sand to hide the litter. It looked clean around 7:00 AM. A delicious breeze made the 100% humidity mixed with the 91-degree temperature tolerable. The sun was strong, so I worked on my tan line every day, forgetting about the torrential black cloud back home.

It was a great escape.

The group of people my new boss knew there was impressive. A designer friend showed us some projects he was working on. An old Spanish hacienda in the "Caleta" part of town where John Wayne once owned a home. A modern one built into the hillside of the Las Brisas community. And a condo in a high-rise building in the center of the bay. We were invited to cocktail parties in homes owned by Norte Americanos (and back then there were a lot of them). We dined at some very unusual restaurants. Every meal was served outside. Our first night there we ate Chinese with delicious, sweet sour sauces!

Frank had a client whom we met the day after we arrived. Gertrude was a snowbird from Chicago. Sometimes during the winter she'd stay in her penthouse in a mid-rise building near our hotel. Condominio Camelia y Magnolia. Her home was beautifully furnished with unusual artwork and lots of bright, multi-colored fabrics. Magenta colored bougainvillea, palm trees and a stunning life-size female sculpture embellished the enormous terrace overlooking the bay.

As soon as we entered the condo, Frank insisted on rearranging the furniture, moving the artwork and visiting a nursery to purchase healthier looking plants for the veranda. I drove the four of us. Minerva, the housekeeper who spoke no English came too in a small Renault with a clutch and rusted floor.

In the short time we spent with this gracious lady, I learned a lot about art, antiques and style. (She had great style.). However, Frank's behavior disappointed her. When I was not with them, he spoke harshly to her. For no reason. About nothing.

He could be that way.

Within a few years, Gertrude would become a very dear friend of mine. We traveled back and forth to Acapulco together. We shopped together, went to museums and the theatre together. We dined together. She continued my exposure to the finer things in life.

When we returned from our escape, Frank continued to pester Terry about the lawsuit until he finally conceded and prepared the legal documents required to sue Paul. Courtesy of these two men, I got the equivalent of a Northwestern University Pritzker Law School education with a minor in what constitutes a counter suit which Paul's lawyer filed.

One evening, after most of our office building's tenants left for the day, someone broke into the Byron, Wiltgen and Associates space. The burglar was ever so careful not to leave telltale signs. The locks were changed, but a 6-inch painter's scraping blade apparently pried open the latch. Did he wear gloves to conceal fingerprints? Or switch on the lights enabling passengers on the El train to notice?

What do you think?

The next morning, when Rhonda and Paul discovered their checkbook, accounts receivable and payable ledgers missing, they suspected moi.

Can you believe that?

Jerry buzzed two uniformed policemen into our office suite when they rang the buzzer. A brief explanation for their appearance made it clear they suspected I was the one who broke into my former office across the hall.

The one that still had my name on the door.

I was read my rights, arrested, and hauled off to jail. They even handcuffed me before parading me down the hallway, into the elevator, and out of the building. Like I was some sort of criminal. Rhonda and Paul were the criminals taking advantage of someone who wasn't 20 years old. After hours of interrogation in a dirty police station, looking like it badly needed Frank and I to better it's appearance, I was allowed one phone call.

"Your life really is a mess, isn't it?" Mom responded when I phoned home. "What are you going to do now?"

That wasn't exactly what I needed to hear. I was hoping she would tell me not to worry; she'd be there as soon as possible.

But Mom had her own problems (my dad), and she couldn't think straight. Instead, Frank once again came to the rescue. He charged in, wearing that flashy, very ostentatious Tanuki coat, demanding to speak with the commander of the police district. After throwing around the names of judges, a district attorney he knew, and the Pritzkers—he told him my history. He had my story memorized. The commander and arresting police officers agreed my partners were scum but said it would be better for me in court if I returned the goods, IF I HAD THE GOODS, which, I must confess, I did. So I did.

That is how I came to believe the only good partner is a dead one!

Months later, my felony case was heard in court. My family was there to support me. After the judge reprimanded the Byron's for taking advantage of an extremely young man, the case was dismissed without talk of a settlement. Frank thanked the judge whom he knew personally.

I wanted to be bought out and the company name changed. But that is something known as a civil suit, which usually comes in an expensive gray Merino wool.

During the hearing, while everyone was in court, someone broke into the Byron, Wiltgen office. Again. This time, whoever it was absconded with the furniture and office equipment. Someone with a truck. I could not be blamed. I just had a Cadillac.

After court, my parents, Cindy, Frank, and I were on our way to lunch when we saw Rhonda and Paul exiting the office building. Their discovery of the second, more impressive theft, was apparent on their faces. After that the Byron, Wiltgen and

Associates office closed. Rhonda stopped providing interior design services working exclusively for the friendly skies of United.

My association with Frank represented a pivotal period in my personal life and career. Like an ancient Roman in good standing, he exposed me to sexual activities between men. Two thousand years ago this included an older male taking a younger one under his wing with all that entailed. Even though I hadn't previously felt attracted to men there were no conflicts. No guilt or shame. Oddly enough, I was okay with having physical relations with either sex. That way, I could easily give up men or women without having to give up dating.

At one time I was so in love with Leana I wanted to marry her. Willy, my best friend at the time, talked sense into me, declaring I was far too young. Then came Rhonda, the extreme opposite of Leana. I was infatuated with her even though, honestly, I knew it wouldn't last. I was way too young and not nearly successful enough. There was no way I could provide the lifestyle to which she was accustomed. For her, I was a diversion. For me, she was a superb instructor. Sexuality is a complex synthesis of standards, attractions, sensations, lust, love and fantasy.

OR is that what design is?

As an uber successful, professional designer, Frank's domineering influence represented a finishing school, elevating me to an entirely new level of ideas, creativity, and affluent clients. Under Frank's wing provided me the opportunity to go behind the doors of some of the most prestigious buildings Willy and I only admired from the seats of our 10-speeds.

What emerged was the creative excellence and superior quality in design, styling and craftsmanship that became the hallmark of John Robert Wiltgen Design, Inc.

Frank's family seemingly accepted his sexual orientation. His elegant mother, diplomatic sister and corporate executive brother were amiable and open minded. It didn't matter to any of them whether he liked boys or girls, men or women. I learned a lot about tolerance and acceptance from their examples. We all liked each other. That's what mattered.

Those who succeed learn something new every day. I learned Frank was bi-polar, although I certainly did not know his mercurial temperament with profound mood swings had a name. He could be sweet, tender and compassionate one minute and as angry as three Chinese whores with their hair on fire the next.

He was still lamenting his former boyfriend of six years who moved to Houston to manage the Revillon Fur Salon, so he needed a distraction. That was me. In the office he criticized my every move in front of Jerry, vendors and even clients. In the first six months of my employment with him, I wanted to quit so many times, but worried how that would look on my resume. The debacle with Byron, Wiltgen and Associates? Then the one with Frank? I did not want current and potential clients to think me unreliable. Deciding to stay for at least one whole year, I took his criticisms like a man and learned all I could.

In mid-December of 1980, I finally gave Frank my two weeks' notice. It was hard for me. I was sad and afraid, but mostly, exhausted from his mood swings. I told him I appreciated all he'd done for me, but felt it was time for both of us to move on.

He was livid! His raging temper hit overdrive.

After packing up my desk and leaving his office for the last time, Frank phoned my mother and outed me to her using extremely profane language and graphic descriptions of my sexual encounters with him and other men. Overnight he transformed into the asshole Mr. Hyde. There were no other men. That mood swing turned the eventful year I spent with him into something crude and disgusting.

Of course, Mom was devastated. I WAS DEVASTATED. The vulgar foulmouthed stories she heard from Frank frightened her and broke her heart. As a devout Catholic, Mom lived a relatively sheltered life for a 44-year-old mother of four. Until that phone call which changed her life forever.

Her oldest was living in the fast lane on the speedway of life. Afraid I might die tomorrow I couldn't help it. Years would pass before Mom would understand my choices. The indiscretions with Mrs. Robinson were inconceivable to her, but Frank's denigrations were depraved. Worse than Mom's mortal sin for her divorcing Dad, she feared I was going to hell and prayed for God's forgiveness.

When I came home that evening everyone was asleep. I let myself in the front door and went down to my dungeon. A spider was spinning a new web in the corner of my dark and lonely bedroom. I hadn't been there in a while. A plain white envelope lay on top my bedspread.

Dare I open it?

I couldn't handle any more trauma. I was tired and wanted to sleep for 100 years like what's her name. Sitting down on the edge of my bed, my lack of self-control made me open the sealed envelope. Mom felt I was a disgrace to our family and did not want me around my brother and sisters. Demanding I move out, she did not know what was wrong with me but feared it might be contagious!

Never meaning to hurt anyone, I also could not lie. The newest truth was out, although I wasn't quite sure what the newest truth was. Personally, I didn't identify as homosexual. I hardly knew what that meant. Maybe bisexual. What did I know? Claiming I knew everything, in one crashing moment it became obvious I still had a lot to learn. I didn't feel I was doing anything wrong, just something different. I had always been different.

Working with clients, designing the spaces they lived in, many were afraid of doing something different. That's why they needed me. To help them decide to take that step and enjoy something extraordinary.

The following morning, when I woke, the house was empty. I made my bed, packed up my drugs, some clothes and left without a good-bye. It was nothing to laugh about, so I cried.

DIAGNOSIS
DIABETES

During the summer between my second and third grade, my family moved to Arlington Heights. Mom and Dad bought my grandparent's house. It had a wood-burning fireplace made of chunky rough-cut stones in its carpeted living room.

Wall-to-wall carpet was the rage back then.

Cindy and I were enrolled in the rather respected Our Lady of the Wayside School. The Catholic Church prides itself on odd parish names guaranteed to make people think one is joking and ask, "You went…where?"

My family is very religious. Mom went to Catholic schools from the first grade through high school and so did all her sisters. She even wanted to be a nun, but my grandpa wouldn't let her. We went to church every Sunday. As a little boy, I could recite almost the entire mass, word for word, unless the mass was in Latin. I even wanted to be a priest when I grew up. The problem is, I am strong-minded and at the time my handicap was being left-handed. Sister Mary Holy Water continually rapped that hand with a ruler to make me use my right one. One day, I grabbed it and hit her back.

My defiance was so unforgiveable I was thrown out of the Catholic grade school the third day of the third week of third grade. So was Cindy. She was in first grade and a totally different room, but we were considered fruit from the same tree.

The priest quoted Mathew 7:17 "…a bad tree bears bad fruit."

Cindy was less independent than I, so the expulsion was traumatic for her. With such a disgrace she wondered how she would ever get dates when she was older.

But honestly, getting kicked out improved our lives. We went to Park School, the public one across the street and loved it. Not only was their playground better, but we didn't have to go to church every day. I was a good left-handed student there getting A's. To keep us from becoming total heathens, Mom enrolled us in Saturday catechism classes where she became a volunteer teacher.

Praise Jesus.

So my childhood was rather ordinary until I started feeling not so good.

At first Mom thought I had the flu. I kept throwing up, had a fever, drank lots of water, urinated constantly and was crabby. That wasn't like me.

"Rest. You need rest," my nurse (Mom) kept saying.

So, I rested and within five or six weeks lost 25 pounds. In third grade I was a tubby little boy weighing in at a whopping 90 pounds. (The average 8-year-old boy weighed 57 pounds.) What can I say? I like food and that was before America got super-sized.

Finally, Mom took me to our family doctor. Dr. Schell delivered me and gave me the snip. After my latest examination, he ordered mom take me directly to Holy Family Hospital. A few days before Christmas we learned I had juvenile onset diabetes which was then and still is incurable. The doctor didn't sugarcoat his diagnosis preparing mom and dad for the worst. My body was not producing insulin needed to remove glucose from my bloodstream. This robbed my heart, liver and other organs of energy. My muscle and natural stores of fat were shrinking while glucose pooled in my bloodstream, pulling fluid from the tissue. Dehydrating me. As a kid, I really felt awful.

An IV drip provided fluid. Needing three nurses to hold me down was a source of pride. I screamed as I fought them. Might have even called them names. Not very nice ones. I cried. A lot. I didn't want to be in the hospital. I wanted to be home for Christmas with Ray, Cindy and our cousins. Then I learned my brother and sister were sent to Tomahawk with Grandma and Grandpa Niemec, so both my parents had time for me. That only made things worse. I'd never been to Wisconsin's north woods in the winter. I wanted to go. Why couldn't I go?

It was the first Christmas in our new home and, as sick as I was, I already hung the stockings on the fireplace mantel. Now, how would Santa know where to find me? Was I still going to get presents? Did he think I did something bad?

Every night, during visiting hours, aunts and uncles came. They tried to cheer me up by bribing me with gifts. That didn't work. I didn't want their stupid gifts. I wanted to go home. They left shaking their heads. On their way out I heard them whisper to Mother, saying "It's too bad…It's such a shame…What are you going to do? We have to pray…"

My life suddenly changed. I felt cursed. Fearful. My parents were afraid, although they tried not to show it. I overheard doctors say my life would be shorter than my siblings. I could go blind, develop kidney disease OR have a leg chopped off. I'll probably die of heart disease or a stroke. And a Merry Fucking Christmas to you too!

Every day, before each meal and at bedtime, I had to pee in a cup, which was tested to see how much sugar was in my urine. This was the only way the doctors and nurses could make me better. The results of the tests determined what happened next…four to six times a day. This was way before modern day glucometers, which measure glucose in our blood stream much more accurately than peeing in a cup. "Testing" my piss. Getting out the eye dropper. Sucking up some piss. Putting 25 drops of urine in a test tube and adding the blue tablet.

No. Not Viagra. You all have a one-track mind!

Watching the mixture of urine and the tablet turn color provided a range of how much glucose was in my urine. Was it normal? Was it moderate? Was it too high? But that was not all…

For the rest of my life I would need insulin. By injection. Every single day. Perhaps a mixture of more than one kind. Regular was the fast-acting type. Lente was slower and longer lasting. A little bit of this and a lot more of that. All determined by my pee. The doctors and nurses tried to figure out how much insulin my body required. Fifty-four and a half years later they are still trying to perfect my dosage.

The hospital imprisoned me for 10 days and I HATED IT. It seemed like forever. The three other kids in our sterile room hidden behind lots of curtains didn't stay nearly that long. One by one they went home before Christmas. For Santa. But they wouldn't let me leave until I could give myself "the shot". Mom and Dad had to learn too. We practiced using a non-disposable glass syringe on an orange. The nurse watched. Someone, probably a cannibal like the infamous Dr. Lecter, decided an orange peel was close to the firmness of a human thigh.

Much worse than all that, though, was the food. I had to go on a "diet". No more cake. No more candy. No more kolaczkis, my favorite Polish cookies. No more sugar-coated cereals for breakfast. How I loved Frosted Flakes. I can still see Tony the Tiger with his bowl declaring "They're great"! When whole milk was poured over the cereal—it was like dessert. And who doesn't like dessert?

Food portions had to be precise. We were told to use a measuring cup. Meat needed to be weighed on a scale AFTER it was cooked. Something about bread exchanges and fruit exchanges and fat exchanges and meat exchanges. I could eat all the free foods I wanted (raw or blanched vegetables), although they weren't what I wanted.

Today, Diabetics are taught to count carbs and the treatment of and survival with diabetes is significantly better, but in 1967, the life expectancy of an insulin dependent diabetic born in 1959 was not to exceed 40. Twenty-seven years less than someone without the disease.

Why me, I continually wondered? I was only 8-years old and already hated my life.

CRAZY
WORLD

When my 10 days were up, I went home to live a life that would never be the same.

The first morning, when I injected myself, the needle went right in. FAST. Like the nurses showed me. Every time after that, I hesitated and then slowly pushed the needle in. It would have been easier if I did it faster, but I could not. I cannot. The thought hurts much worse than the actual shot.

To this day I close my eyes and look away when someone in a movie gets one. Especially for the close ups. I love horror films. People getting stabbed in the shower, or chased with a chain saw, or Zombies walking the streets of London, but I cannot watch a drug addict shooting up heroin or Dr. Doug Ross, played by George Clooney on the TV show *ER*, sticking a needle in a patient's vein. It is too close to home.

In those days, the glass syringe was sterilized after each use. Boiled in a pot of water. Mom was a good nurse and gave me shots all the time, rotating sites. When she stuck me, I hardly felt it. She was much better than me. Dad stunk at giving me the shot and avoided it like the plague. That made me think he didn't care.

Then came disposable syringes. No more standing by a pot of boiling water. Most insulin dependent diabetics still use them today. Some people even reuse them because the cost of all the supplies is quite expensive and if you don't have insurance you're screwed.

I would use the "f" word, which is more fitting, but I am trying to keep this clean.

Nowadays, some diabetics wear insulin pumps, a small pocket-sized machine which enables insulin to be delivered into the body automatically. It can also deliver additional doses whenever needed, before meals, for instance.

I wear a Medtronic 670 G. It has been either plugged into my ass or stomach since 2001. It is much easier than filling a syringe three or four times daily and provides diabetics much better management of the disease. My Hemoglobin A1 C test results, which measures the amount of glucose in your bloodstream over a three-month period, have improved tremendously since I started using it.

After first being diagnosed, I was so miserable. I couldn't understand why this happened to me. I hated God. How could He allow this? I hated my parents for making me—however they did that. I hated my brother and sister because now I was different. I was so jealous. I hated them and everybody and everything.

However, I discovered some sort of relief. Within a short amount of time, I reasoned, if I was going to be miserable everyone else would be miserable too.

The logic of an 8-year-old.

Somehow, I'd make them miserable. Why should they be happy? I wanted to be happy.

I didn't want to go to school. I had this disease. Diabetes. What would my classmates say when they found out? There was no way I was going to church on Sundays. I was SO pissed at God. If there even was a God. Which was hard to believe.

I didn't want to go to the brand-new Woodfield Mall and watch everyone eating food I couldn't have. Cotton candy. Hot caramel corn. Donuts. Or the movie theaters with all that fake buttered popcorn and chocolate malted milk balls.

For the same reasons, I didn't want to go to other people's houses. Like my grandparent's. Despite my newly acquired hatred for everyone, I loved all my grandparents dearly and didn't think they had anything to do with me getting this disease. However, at their homes I could not eat what everyone else did. I couldn't drink what they were drinking. It wasn't fair.

Diet this. Sugar free that. Tab. Fresca. Saccharine.

Mom shopped differently. Cooked differently. And, in her defense, she made everyone else eat differently too. Said we were all going to be healthier because of me. No more Twinkies or Little Debbie's or her pineapple upside-down cake. She was a good baker.

Back then, we were taught I could have a piece of fruit. An apple or half a banana. Today we know most fruits quickly turn into simple sugar and should be avoided altogether.

By treating everyone the same Mom tried to make me feel better, but did that work? No. Not at all. I couldn't be bought. I became a rebel and would remain one most of my life.

When it was time to go to one of our relatives' homes, I would run into my bedroom (shared with Ray), lock the door, throw myself on my bed, and cry.

Knock. Knock.

"What?" I replied as wretchedly as I knew how.

"Come on," mom pleaded. "It's time to go…"

"I don't care. I don't want to go."

"Of course you do. You just don't know it yet," she tried to be patient with me, but I ruined it for everyone; so badly they all stayed home. Mom and Dad would fight. Cindy and Baby Ray would cry. We were one big tragically unhappy family. All because of me and diabetes.

Once, in church, (the same one that kicked Cindy and me out of its school) when it was so quiet, probably right after the priest said, "Let us pray," I passed out. Mom cried as Father carried me down the aisle like a roll of carpeting.

Baby Ray asked OUT LOUD, "Is he dead? Is he dead?"

Suddenly, everyone stopped praying to look at us. Some of the parishioners thought I was possessed. If I could have, I would have stuck my tongue out at them. That might have made me feel good. But I couldn't. I was a goner.

This happened a lot. At home. On the playground. In the car when my Mom was driving. Even in church.

At the ER (not the one with Dr. Ross) they always asked so many stupid questions. What's your name? Do you know what day it is? Where do you live? The doctors worried my unconscious seizures might be a sign of something wrong with my brain while my parents insisted I needed anything with a lot of sugar. Then, because I got something with a lot of sugar my blood glucose would spike, I'd need a dose of Regular insulin (the fast-acting kind) to lower the glucose to a safe level.

My school health incidents scared the b'jesus out of my classmates and teachers. It scared the heck out of me too. After a while everyone learned I needed orange juice to return to the living. The entire rhythm of my existence was set to the rise and fall of my glucose. Most of my classmates thought I was a freak, but in fourth grade one of the jocks befriended me. I agreed to teach him how to draw and he taught me how to play baseball. He could always tell when I needed the candy in my pocket and made me eat it, even if it was melted and gooey.

A BETTER ME

My youngest sister Regina was born Friday, October 2, 1970. Her name was a combination of our parents first names: Ray and Jean. The stork delivered her to the hospital eight years after Baby Ray and he was thrilled. He could now pass his "baby" title onto the youngest member of our family.

When Regina came home everyone took care of her. Loving her. Feeding her. Rocking her to sleep. Changing her diapers. By then diapers were disposable so no one had to wash them.

Yuck! Can you imagine? Washing dirty diapers?

Before long Regina's crib went in the room Cindy previously had to herself. That did not go over well with my 10-year-old sister. In Regina's defense, she had nothing to do with it. At four months, even if my parents asked her if she wanted to be Cindy's roommate, I'm sure she'd be too stunned to reply.

Not wanting to hear all the crying that took place in the middle of the night, I moved to the basement. There was a crappy bathroom down there no one else used, so I took ownership. Dad and I remodeled the below grade level. It was one of the few things we did together as father and son. We framed the foundation walls with 2x4's, added insulation, a layer of Visqueen, concrete board and then covered that with a brick veneer. Z-Brick. We thought it looked tasteful, but what did we know? Nothing. I am sure that behind all our work, the concrete walls were, in time, covered in black mold.

My bedroom was just below Cindy and Regina's. It came with two walls of bleached, tongue and groove paneling on the two interior walls that was there when my grandpa bought the house. Dad and I installed Z-brick on the two exterior ones. We made five decorative arched recesses in the brick veneered walls into which we glued blue, and I mean bright blue, indoor/outdoor carpet.

I am not kidding. If anyone suggested that design idea today I would shoot them.

To me, back then, it looked cool, and all my friends thought we were monied. Eventually, I hung my artwork in each arch, which was even more cool, but that was after Phase 1 when I used black lights to illuminate psychedelic glow-in-the-dark posters.

My favorite poster featured a green gremlin-type character with one leg up on a rock while flipping the bird and a phrase "this one's for you…" When Mom saw it thumbtacked on the carpeted arch, she did a double take, froze, and quickly tore it down and threw it away. She said I was much too young for a poster like THAT. The next day I bought another and kept my door shut.

The concrete floor was finished with red, white, and blue Congoleum vinyl flooring in anticipation of our country's 200-year anniversary. Dad and I created the custom pattern. My decorating career had just begun though I didn't know it.

My basement also included an office area with a big metal executive desk and file cabinets. I love file cabinets and claimed that space as mine too. Mom bought an old-fashioned Under-wood typewriter for me at a garage sale. I wrote stories and plays, and before long I was the editor of the South Junior High school newspaper. If you don't think that got me into a lot of trouble you are *wrong*. When I wrote and published a story about a music teacher whom I wasn't particularly fond, the principal immediately relieved me of my pro-bono job, ending my career in journalism.

When Regina was two, she became extremely sick and had to go to the hospital where mom had a job preparing and sterilizing surgical trays for $4.00 an hour. Our family needed the money. Regina had the flu. Just like me when I was diagnosed with diabetes. I prayed all day and night to the God at whom I was still so pissed. I did not want Regina to become diabetic too. Even though I was busy making the whole world miserable, I loved my little sister and would do anything for her. Hoping He was listening, I begged God to please not let Regina have diabetes. In return, I bargained, I would stop making everyone unhappy.

Mom came home late at night after visiting Regina in her hospital room. She looked so sad; her eyes bloodshot from the tears she shed during her walk home. Back then, we had one car and Father was rarely around when Mom needed a ride. They were not living in domestic bliss.

Regina did not develop juvenile-onset diabetes. Thank God. I made a truce with Him, promising to be a better person, take care of myself and try not to make anyone else's life miserable anymore. Unless they deserved it!

THE
ODD COUPLE

Repeatedly loitering at a sad excuse for a strip mall in downtown Arlington Heights, I met Willy. He worked at a paint store selling wallpaper, picture frames, art supplies and paint. His boss was an older woman, Margaret Donahugh.

Dr. Lidge, our family dentist, had an arrangement with the pharmacy in Dunton Court, giving prescriptions for a free ice cream cone or sandwich each time our teeth were cleaned (the perfect snack for an already out of control juvenile diabetic). I rode my bicycle to the pharmacy immediately after each dental visit somehow ending up at the paint store. I loved the smell of the vinyl wallpaper books.

I annoyed Willy enough to learn his name, where he lived, finally convincing him we should ride bikes together. I did a lot of bike riding then. Not because the exercise was good for me, although it was, but because I was too young to drive a car. Those days kid's mothers did NOT chauffeur their offspring around the way they do today. If we wanted to go to the library or movie theater we had to walk or ride our bikes or not go and instead play in our backyard. Fortunately, Willy was old enough to drive and had a brand-new yellow Camaro with a bike rack.

I was excited about becoming a high school freshman. He was going to be a freshman too, in college. He lived at home, went to college, worked at the paint store and was the night manager of the movie theater in town. That came with some benefits. Like free popcorn and admission which means we rarely missed a movie. He was my mentor and I mean that in the least sarcastic way.

To ingratiate myself to both Willy (short for William) and Mrs. Donahugh (she said I could call her Margaret), I would buy them ice cream cones, too. Even though I did not know what ingratiate meant, Willy and I became fast friends.

We were like the odd couple. Willy's family was rich as in "very". Mine was not. His family owned a large seafood distributorship. My family worked for people who worked for people who owned businesses. Willy lived with his parents in a beautiful condominium development that had a pond, water features and manicured landscaping. I chopped down the cherry tree in our backyard with an axe leaving the stump sticking out of the ground for years. I did, I cannot tell a lie.

Willy's home was filled with fancy furniture. Carved. Gold leafed. Marble tops. Damask patterned fabrics with plastic slip covers. I had never seen anything like that before. Grandpa Niemec's house in Park Ridge was furnished by John M. Smythe Co., but it didn't come close to this version of 1970's elegance.

Our house had a big backyard and when we let the dogs, Topsy (an old black lab) and Heidi (a sleek, energetic Weimaraner) in, they often brought live baby rabbits with them. Those two dogs were so proud when they'd open their mouths and the bunnies would jump out and sprint around the house. Much to their delight and ours. Not Mothers.

Willy was a good dresser. Even when mixing cans of paint or drying down custom color samples on a wooden stirring stick, he always looked professional. His influence prompted me to throw away my blue and white denim train engineers cap I wore through most of junior high.

Both of Willy's brothers lived downtown so he was quite familiar with getting around Chicago. On his day off we would take our bicycles to the big city and ride for miles. I loved it. Up and down the lakefront I often ran into other cyclists or joggers because I was too busy admiring the combination of old and new buildings on Lake Shore Drive. I couldn't begin to imagine what the inside of these condos looked like.

Continuing through Lincoln Park, which parallels Lake Michigan for seven miles, we would stop for a hot dog or two when I needed to eat. Originally a cemetery, it is the second most visited city park after New York City's Central Park. Past the zoo and several museums, we'd end up at the Gold Coast's picture-perfect Astor Street to admire the magnificent 19th-century historic stone mansions hidden in the shadows of newly erected luxury high-rise buildings.

I soon became intimate with a city that, ultimately, has been extremely good to me. Willy was generous with his time and knowledge of Chicago and its founding fathers. For that I am forever grateful.

Around my 14th birthday, a friend from junior high helped me get a job at Eddie's Lounge—not quite a fast-food place—but not a fine dining establishment either. He said I had to be 16. So, I WAS 16.

My next two years were spent washing dishes, breading chicken, washing dishes, breading fish, washing dishes, bussing tables, washing dishes and bringing up cases of bottled beer from the walk-in cooler in the cellar. I was very proud I could carry three cases up the cellar stairs all at once.

I worked three or four nights a week from five to nine. Thursday nights we breaded 300 pounds of fish for Friday's fish fry. Friday, we worked until 11. When I got home, I smelled so fishy Mom wouldn't let me in the front door of our house. Instead, she made me go down the concrete stairs in the garage to the basement laundry room where I stripped everything off and threw the stinky apparel into the washing machine.

At Eddie's Lounge, we served a lot of fried food and so I ate a lot of fried food. Fried fish. Fried chicken. French fries with tons of regular ketchup. It was okay for my pocketbook, but not for my diabetes.

IN A NEW YORK MINUTE

After Frank outed me to Mom, I moved out of my family's house for a season. I stayed with a friend and resuscitated John Robert Wiltgen Design, Inc. Some clients of the defunct Byron, Wiltgen and Associates, and two of Frank's asked me to help them finish their homes.

The first six months of my relaunch in 1981 kept me frantically busy. I was a one-man show and did everything. Drawings by hand. 3-D renderings finished with acrylics, markers, and colored pencils. Invoices, purchase orders and all the bookkeeping accompanying my small business. My prior work experience came in handy. I shopped for furniture, fabric, art and antiques for my projects. Thank you, Frank, for all you taught me. I met with clients. Tried to find new business. Prepared "Letters of Agreement" for every job. Developed a biography and postcards with photos of my work for marketing purposes.

In my spare time, I tried to be a better diabetic. What that meant was, after speeding through the last four years of my life without a doctor or blood test, I finally found an internist to keep tabs on me.

***

In February, I received a shocking phone call from guess who? The former Mrs. Byron. My answering service took her call. I wasn't sure I wanted to speak with her, but my male curiosity got the best of me. The conversation began with small talk. She was no longer in the design business and heard I left Frank's employ. She had a referral for me. But first...

Okay. Here it comes, I thought.

...I must promise not to reveal my age. OK. That was not what I was thinking but it was hard to escape the curse of my youth. I agreed. Anything to make a buck.

A friend of hers was marketing a high-rise rental building planned for a potentially up and coming neighborhood. On Michigan Avenue, though far south of the Magnificent Mile her friend needed a designer to help with—well EVERYTHING. The lobby, corridors, rental offices, models, party room, health club, even the laundry room. She gave me his contact information and said he was expecting my call. After a few more trivial pleasantries, our conversation ended.

Still in awe when I phoned Rhonda's friend, he confirmed I came highly recommended. Why was she being nice now? But I didn't waste any time trying to solve that mystery. People try and never discover the correct answer. What's the point?

As per Rhonda's instructions, I did not tell him my age and was immediately engaged to design all the interiors for 1212 S. Michigan Avenue. It was an enormous commission for any design firm, especially one owned and operated by a 22-year-old.

I immediately hired two assistants. The finished product led to a project in Atlanta by the same development firm. Combined with the homes I was working on I was quite busy and off to a great restart.

***

Eventually, Mom and I kissed and made up. Not quite sure how we should handle our traumatic past, we downplayed the whole Frank scenario and her remarrying Dad. She chose not to ask any questions or offer much information. Neither did I. There was no drama. Her broken heart mended itself and my spirit was restored. We both tried to understand the other and be happy in the moment. The reconciliation brought a welcomed sense of relief to our entire family.

With Dad's return came a small, single mast sailboat which everyone enjoyed on sunny breezy weekends. We played a game trying to get the sail to lay just above the water as we sat on the high side of the boat. If the sail and mast dipped beneath the surface of the lake it would tip. That was our idea of fun.

I often brought my friend Gera-Lynd with me. As the assignment editor for a major television station's news program, she always came with the most interesting stories. Babies thrown out of windows. A woman raped in a changing room of one of Chicago's major department stores. The body of a man found in the alley of Boystown. Wearing combat boots, she would drive to my folk's house in her old beat-up car sporting numerous bullet holes which added to the authenticity of her stories.

To make her appear somewhat graceful, she asked me to teach her how to dance. That was no easy assignment. We went from one disco to another as they were still in vogue. When she was ready, we attended various social events and black-tie charity balls together. My parents were thrilled. Seemed I had outgrown my interest in men. Little did they know, when the two of us went out Gera-Lind was deciding on men for me, and I was eyeing women for her. It was a game we played which neither one of us were very good at, so at the end of the evening, I would drop her off at her parents' home and then take myself back to Arlington Heights.

I finally decided on my preference of men over women. My personal distorted impression was men were stronger and I suspected there would come a time in my life when I would need someone as tough as me to help me survive. However, I must admit to befriending a lot of emotionally strong, business savy, powerful women too.

Moving back to my basement bedroom I wanted to live downtown. However, having rented an office near the Mart I was worried about overextending myself. How much money would John Robert Wiltgen Design, Inc. need to survive the start-up years? For that reason, I asked a crazy Realtor friend of mine to sell my condo. Despite the improvements and high interest rates, I made a few scheckles which came in handy. After that Lucille began showing me three-flats which, she proposed, I could live in while my tenants paid the mortgage and taxes.

A friend of mine, also named John, and I bought a red brick three-flat scheduled for demolition in a poor Chicago neighborhood called Bucktown. That name was inspired by goats stowed by immigrants in their basements for milk. We knew each other since our dishwashing fishbreading days together at Eddie's Lounge. The building was cheap, $27,000, probably because of all the work it needed. Less than what I paid for my condo. Interest rates were more than eighteen percent. Lucille professionally advised it was more money to deduct from our income taxes.

The building was falling apart and boarded up. Occasionally homeless people camped there. I went to building court by myself to contest the demolition explaining to a judge our plans to improve the property. He asked if I was a lawyer.

It needed everything. A new roof, windows, electrical service, plumbing, kitchens and baths, furnaces and air conditioning. Drywall, doors, door casings, baseboards, and carpeting. Maybe crown moldings depending on if there was any money left. Light fixtures and locks.

Thank God we had no idea what that meant in terms of dollars and cents. Otherwise, we would never have bought it. Our inexperience made it affordable.

The first floor, once a butcher shop, was converted to a two-bedroom apartment with 14-foot ceilings. There were two more two-bedroom apartments on the floors above. In all three, the bedrooms were tiny, but the living, dining rooms and kitchens were spacious. There was a rooftop smokehouse, typical for buildings that formerly housed butcher shops. John and I planned to live in the third-floor apartment. We wanted to convert the smokehouse to our office with a great view of the Chicago skyline. We concocted plans for a rooftop deck.

One weekend, bored with doing all the heavy lifting, John and I decided to have a "bring your own crowbar" party. We had a grill on the rooftop and bought some cheap outdoor furniture. Even Gertrude showed up from her elegant East Lake Shore Drive co-op with a pink jeweled hammer. We got absolutely nothing done but everyone had a great time exploring the three floors and roof and asked to be invited back when we were finished.

I had a huge schoolboy crush on John. Having known him for a long time, he knew as much about me as my family. And my family always treated him like family. He was handsome, hard-working, and often helped me forget about my fear of going blind. John was kind but strong. In our building, he would guide me up and down the stairs; made sure I didn't fall; and was keenly aware of my need to eat if there was to be no passing out consequences. We were invited to dinner parties at friends' homes, some very gay friends, with whom he seemed comfortable. We shared most of my clients. Though my fondness for him soared I was afraid of ruining our friendship.

Around that time, Leana returned from Arizona. She had not been home for several years; missed her grandma's funeral (she was in some jungle with one of her professors not to be found until gram was not only dead but buried). With Rhonda now out of my life, she wondered where she fit in. I didn't tell her about Frank or my manly inclinations.

We had Leana's former college friends in common. Sue and Cynthia. Sue worked for a crazy art dealer friend of mine. Cynthia tended bar at Harry's Café on Rush Street. After majoring in fashion design, Cynthia Rowley became the famous global lifestyle designer.

One evening, Leana and I were invited to a party at their place. They lived in an old brownstone at 15 E. Pearson between State Street and Michigan Avenue. Someone suggested we make "pot" brownies. We ran right into the vintage kitchen and found the brownie mix. Leana was given the baggie of grass. It took us three minutes to add water and stir. And stir and stir and stir.

We dumped the mix into a greased brownie pan and licked the bowl and spoon. Nothing went to waste. We sniffed at the oven as the brownies baked. When finished, we were eager to try them. Leana and I sampled the edibles immediately each eating one. Nothing happened so we helped ourselves to another. We delivered the rest to the group in the living room. Then BAM.

It hit me like something round from outer space. Before I knew it, I was 20 or 30 feet above the worn hardwood floors. Everyone sat on the floors staring up at me. It was scary. Leana was gone. I kept yelling "Where is Leana? Where is she?" They all laughed.

I managed to find her in a bedroom curled up on the bed. I flew into the room, landed on the bed and crawled up next to her. "Are you okay?" I asked slowly.

She shook her head no.

"What's wrong?" more slowly.

"I'm afraid," she responded.

"Afraid of what?" even slower.

"You!"

"Me?" I pointed to my chest in very slow motion.

She shook her head, then tried to hide in the pillows.

I raced back to the parlor where everyone was still laughing. What was so funny? Suddenly I had the munchies, so I glided into the kitchen to see what I could find. I ate everything a diabetic shouldn't. Cookies. Cereal. Bread. A banana. My sugar level climbed higher and higher, but I could not control myself.

It was time to leave. Leana was serving communion at her Eastern Orthodox church in the morning. That, I thought, was VERY funny. So did everyone else. We all laughed. And laughed. And laughed. Leana was frightened. She got into the back seat of my car. Still afraid, she didn't express the same amusement as the rest of us.

I didn't get out of my bed for three days. Cynthia and Sue called several times. When I picked up the phone all I could do was laugh. They laughed too. None of us understood how Leana went to church—let alone hand out communion. I've never had anything to do with marijuana since. Never.

A few days later, Cynthia asked if I was interested in driving to New York City. I had to think about it.

In a second, I said "YES".

I volunteered to drive us in my reliable white Ford Granada (I finally got rid of the Cadillac), so she could see a boyfriend and deliver some clothing to two boutiques in the Village. It was my first trip there and, on our departure, I asked, "Do we need a map?"

"No, just go east," she replied while sewing buttons on the outfits she spread out in the back seat. She told me if we ended up in the Atlantic, I went too far!

Six or seven hours into the trip Cynthia slept while we cruised the Pennsylvania Turnpike. I began seeing dark, unnerving spots that were difficult to distinguish from the inky blackness of the night. Headlights of an occasional truck in the opposite lane illuminated the murky spots and thin, wiry streaks, almost like cobwebs, that slowly started to appear in my left eye.

Why wake Cynthia? I didn't want to alarm her. I didn't want to alarm myself. It was nothing said my brain, repeatedly. The condition seemed to improve as I continued driving. The power of a positive mental attitude.

Without incident, we reached New York City the next morning. I dropped Cynthia off somewhere in the Village. Then checked into the vintage Gramercy Park Hotel. It was recently renovated, and she said I would like it. Remodelers turned the original Renaissance Revival interior architecture into something fit for a Brian de Palma thriller. Having just seen his latest movie, *Dressed to Kill*, I thought it best to prop a chair beneath the doorknob to be safe.

Without delay, I jumped into the shower to rinse away the obscure veins which, against the white tile of the bathroom, were far more evident. Pushing up the flesh around my bad eye, I let water wash over it. My mind wandered. No longer able to ignore the issues I was having, a memory I had blocked for years emerged.

I was a kid again, two or three years after my diagnosis, seated at the breakfast table in grouchy Aunt Lil's kitchen. She was talking to my mother about a friend's teenage granddaughter who had juvenile diabetes and became completely blind.

Aunt Lil mentioned the girl's condition in a stage whisper as if the child had slipped into a lesser state of being or the disease was something unholy. Her hushed tone couldn't prevent me from overhearing their conversation. Even though I didn't want to, I heard every word. I wished the girl wasn't blind.

Mom sheltered me from knowing about many of the complications of type 1 diabetes, determined to handle all the worrying. She did a good job. I refused to acknowledge the facts and never thought about that blind girl again.

I live as if there was the diabetic me and the unreal me. Perhaps a condition of split personalities? I much prefer my unreal life, still do to this day. Back then, I dismissed the possibility of losing my sight. Those thoughts washed over me as I stood under the shower spray in my Brian de Palma-esque hotel room. Trying to convince myself many of the spots had been absorbed, their appearance meant I could no longer live-in denial. I had to stop fantasizing a picture-perfect life for myself.

Should I turn around and go home?

No.

I stuck to my plan to explore Manhattan. I spent a day at the Metropolitan Museum of Art examining the Period Rooms, the Egyptian Temple of Dendur and its incredible collection of artifacts. For several days I investigated the variety of "to-the-trade" showrooms in a vast assortment of buildings. I was curious to see if NYC had different/better merchandise than the Chicago Merchandise Mart showrooms. I shopped up and down Fifth Avenue, buying a dress for Mom at Bergdorf Goodman.

Cynthia left a message instructing me to meet for dinner at Elaine's, a popular spot on the Upper East Side. I had no idea what to wear to this "stomping ground of celebrities and wannabees" or what that even meant until I discovered myself sitting next to Cher and Meat Loaf. Meatloaf was not on the menu, but he eyed it intently.

My discovery of New York City ended quickly. While there, I continually pinched myself to make sure it was really happening. Before Cynthia and I could go home we had to deliver her latest fashions to the boutiques in the Village. As we cruised the maze of one-way streets on the lower West Side, she spotted Mary Tyler Moore dining at a sidewalk café.

"STOP!" she ordered. "Park the car. Somewhere. Anywhere. It's time for lunch. Let's see if we can sit at a table close to her. I love Mary Tyler Moore."

So, I parked. And we got a table close to where Mary Tyler Moore sat. We watched her eat and drink her lunch. That was it. We did not say hello. Or ask for an autograph. We just stared. Little did we know then, but Mary was also a type 1 diabetic and years later the Ambassador for the Juvenile Diabetes Research Foundation.

After lunch there was still much to do before leaving Manhattan. But what did I do with the car? Using Mary Tyler Moore as a decoy, maybe Cynthia realized I needed to eat and that is why she ordered me to stop for lunch? I was fine now minus the car. We feared it was stolen. But really, who would want to steal a white Ford Granada with dead bugs masking the windshield? After discovering a NO PARKING sign in a spot that looked vaguely familiar, I asked a police officer where a couple of out-of-towners had to go to retrieve our vehicle.

Hours later, after rescuing the car from the bowels of Manhattan and dropping off the merchandise at the boutiques, it was time to leave the Big Apple. Gassing up, I thoughtlessly got back into my car and drove away from the service station ripping the hose right out of the gas tank. There was smelly, flammable gasoline everywhere.

"Step on it!" Cynthia ordered.

As I did, I spotted an angry attendant in the rear-view mirror chasing us. It reminded me of the days when Leana's mother ran after us, broomstick in hand, as we drove off at 11:00 pm to go discoing on a school night.

DOCTOR
MY EYES

Once Cynthia and I made it home, I dreaded seeing our family eye doctor. The reality of my life was catching up with me. Mom came along. I told him about the cobwebs clouding my vision. He immediately referred us to a specialist he hoped could help. Dr. Carl Fetkenhour was president of the Chicago Ophthalmology Society.

I might not be able to see but that was not an excuse to slack off on the work needed at the building John and I bought. We didn't have enough cash to pay for materials and tradesmen, so we did much of the work ourselves. That was the deal and John depended on me to hold up my end. The work was hard but my version of therapy. I had no idea what would become of my vision.

What to do?

Keep working of course. There was no time to stay home and feel sorry for myself. I made sure of that. It was better for me. Better for my business. And better for our Bucktown 3-flat.

We manhandled 55-gallon drums of garbage down two flights of stairs to the dumpster parked in the street. It took several weekends and numerous dumpsters just to gut the kitchens and baths. We removed some third-floor walls to create a loft-like space before we knew anything about lofts.

On July 21, 1981, Mom drove me to Dr. Fetkenhour's office. She wouldn't let me drive until we saw the specialist. Mom was frightened but kept saying everything would be all right. I *needed* her to believe that. Otherwise she would be devastated.

Coincidentally, the doctor's office was on one of the "professional" floors at Water Tower Place, still one of my favorite Chicago destinations despite the memories of Paul Byron and the 42nd floor.

We were guided into an examination room and a nurse, Brigit, entered. She was a stocky girl, blonde, blue-eyed, who wore a starched white uniform with matching hosiery and shoes. Calm, gentle and kind, Brigit understood my fears. She had experience with the doctor's other patients.

Gently, she dilated my pupils. The lights were off in the windowless room when she asked me to read the chart. It was a struggle. Was it a "V" or an "M"? An "E" or an "F"? An "S" or a "B"? So frustrating.

In came Dr. Fetkenhour. He was a quiet, congenial, older gentleman with a full head of shimmering, silver hair. He reviewed my medical history, then cautiously opened my eyes with two fingers and studied them using a specially lit magnifying glass. Although he put me at ease, the intense penetrating light made my eyes water.

"Look up. Ah ha. Okay, look down. Look left." Then came silent concentration.

What was he thinking?

"Now look straight ahead. Hold it. Look down again." He said he needed to photograph my retinas and optic nerves to learn the location and severity of the damage.

Pointing to a framed, illustrated eye mounted on the wall, he said he suspected I had diabetic retinopathy, which meant blood vessels of the retina were damaged. The floaters and web like images I saw were symptoms of the problem. He ordered tests and then left the room.

Brigit, with her perfect white teeth and perpetually broad smile became my newest best friend. She helped me remain optimistic during terribly frightening times. In simple terms, she explained the next procedure, a *fluorescein angiogram* saying there was nothing to worry about.

That usually means there is something to worry about.

The test uses special dye to study blood flow to the retina and the pigmented vascular layer of the eyeball between its white outer layer and the retina.

Brigit could see the fear of the unknown in my eyes and reassured me. She said I wouldn't feel a thing. "Well, maybe just a little thing."

The IV needle went into a vein on the top of my right hand. Brigit complimented me, "You have GREAT veins." She was good with the IV.

When Fetkenhour returned he placed my head on the chin rest and told me to "open wide". I did. Click, click, click….

The doctor photographed the inside of my eye.

"Hold your eyes open. Don't move John. Good."

After the first group of pictures were taken, Brigit administered fluorescein through the IV. When enough time elapsed, he repeated his commands.

"Hold them open. Don't move. Perfect." The camera's shutter fluttered. Then, he told mom and me to relax while Brigit processed the film.

How do you relax while waiting for bad news?

In the calmness owned only by specialists he confirmed I was experiencing advanced diabetic retinopathy and like half the people with that condition I also had macular edema. This meant fluid and protein deposits were leaking against or under the yellow central area of my retinas, causing them to thicken and swell, especially in my left eye. And that meant...well, it wasn't good.

Mom started crying. Quietly. She didn't want me to be afraid too but out of the corner of my eye I saw her take a tissue to wipe the tears from her face. That broke my heart. Hadn't I put her through enough already?

Diabetic retinopathy has four stages, Dr. Fetkenhour explained. I had Stage Four, known in certain circles as proliferative retinopathy of my left eye.

Lucky me.

Signals sent by the retina for nourishment trigger the growth of new blood vessels. Mine were fragile with thin, delicate walls. From time to time they leaked blood, creating the cobweb effect I saw while driving to New York. Cynthia and I were extremely lucky. With me behind the wheel we could have ended up floating in the Atlantic or worse. The doctor suggested aggressive treatment scheduling me for *laser photocoagulation* several days later.

Back in the car, Mom suggested we pursue a second opinion. She read about a doctor in St. Louis. I did not want to talk to another doctor or to her or anybody else. I wanted this to be over. Despite my confidence in Fetkenhour, panic was starting to set in.

Why is this happening? Why? God, I know I haven't been to church in a long time and there isn't a priest with enough time to listen to my confession. Even the Reader's Digest version. But don't let me go blind. Please.

God: You took good health for granted. That's why. But just for the record... bad things happen to good people. Didn't you read Rabbi Kushner's book? I coached him on it!

As if the possibility was a matter of choice, I decided I was not going blind. Not if I were to continue in my chosen profession.

By my next doctor's visit I learned some jokes (if I were going to laugh, I would make others laugh too) and shared them with the receptionist. The blind and almost blind people sitting in the waiting room were within ear shot. Few of them were happy with my comedy routine which focused mostly on Helen Keller.

To prevent the other patients from overhearing my jokes, Mom and I were quickly escorted to a procedure room where I was seated in a special, leather-covered chair. I was there for laser photocoagulation, hoping it would cauterize my leaky blood vessels. This is a treatment developed in outer space.

Next, as if on cue, Dr. Fetkenhour entered. I wondered if there was a button Bridgit pressed to get him to show up at the right time. After I read the chart, he pressed a lever on the chair putting me flat on my back. Why? He was going to anesthetize the eye. This required a shot straight into my left eye. I could see the needle going in. It freaked me out.

"Don't move," he said. Brigit held my head in her warm hands. She was a strong woman.

I wanted to see him avoid moving as I attempted to stick a needle in his eye.

Then he inserted a thick contact lens containing microscopic mirrors to help him aim the laser beam that would burn and hopefully, seal the bleeding vessels. He tilted the chair upright and gently pushed the chin rest up to my face.

"Now look straight ahead." He put something up to my eye to hold it open. For the next 25 minutes, I saw thousands of flashes of concentrated light beams. My left eye watered. I wanted to blink but couldn't. The leaking blood vessels covered a wide area of my retina. I tried, without success, to count the laser burns as they were applied. There were so many. To my surprise, it didn't hurt, but not knowing if it would work or not was most painful.

When finished, he told me the treatment should slow the progression of diabetic retinopathy. He applied antibiotic ointment and a thick gauze pad over my eye, taped it and sent Mom and me home. We were to return the next day.

When the bandage came off, Fetkenhour seemed pleased with the results. Nevertheless, the danger of the loss of sight hung over my head.

Continuing to build my design business as my vision deteriorated raised many questions. Was I making the right decision? If things got worse, how would I manage? How would I get around? There was neither Lyft nor Uber. How would I write a check? Collect money? Deposit the money? Choose fabrics? I was certifiable.

After this run-in with retinopathy, I was shocked into taking better care of myself. I needed to maintain healthier control of my glucose levels. Several manufacturers created "glucometers," little machines revealing my glucose level by pricking the tip of a finger and placing a drop of blood on the test strip. Until recently, I did that three or four times a day. If my sugar is frighteningly high, like 300 or above, I use my glucometer more often to monitor the situation as I try to bring it down with more insulin.

Before I wore an insulin pump it meant taking more insulin via syringe. Once I started wearing a pump it became much easier to administer more of the hormone, if needed, without an injection. With the pump, it was critical to know my blood glucose.

You never know what you are capable of until you're tested. I was convinced that black cloud followed me everywhere. First it was my love life with Rhonda which fell apart; then, the violent end of Byron, Wiltgen and Associates; after that, my first relationship with a man, a bipolar, twisted man, which concluded theatrically. Like three different Tennessee Williams' plays. I thought that was enough, but I was wrong.

The black cloud was morphing into a twister.

DOWNTOWN

When I started high school (1973) Grandma Wiltgen got a job baking in the cafeteria. She was there every day when I showed up for lunch. Always on the lookout, when she spotted me, her face lit up. Anything I wanted Grandma got for me. More mashed potatoes? Yes, please. Gravy? No, thank you. But could I have some butter? Do you want an apple too? No but how about one of those chocolate chip cookies? Are you supposed to be eating those? Well, Grandma I have gym right after lunch. (I was a very good actor.) Oh okay. Here, why don't you take two…this one is broken!

I didn't worry about the consequences my sweet tooth would present.

Thanks to Paint-Store-Willy, my wardrobe improved which helped impress at least one girl in my social studies class. She was smart and pretty. Blonde hair. Blue eyes. Thin. Crowned Miss Teenage Illinois and Miss Oktoberfest. Jill Ziske was a model. A Wendy Ward model. And, most importantly, she was nice. Really nice.

One day I mustered up the courage to ask her and a girlfriend (also a Wendy Ward model) if they both wanted to go out, hoping it would provide a chance to become better acquainted with them. Well, with Jill actually. And for her to learn about me. I suggested we cut school and take the train downtown. So we did.

We walked to Marc Chagall's new mosaic *the Four Seasons*, in the plaza of what was then the First National Bank. Mom took Ray, Cindy and me to see it the previous summer. It was one of our field trips. The installation was relatively new and received lots of press. Hoping to sound like an art aficionado to the girls, I tried to explain the mosaic and Chagall's effort to bring the skyline image up to date.

When Mom took us to see the mosaic, we dined across the street at the Italian Village. I loved it. The restaurant made me feel like I was on vacation. Designed in 1927, it resembles an actual Italian village with little houses enclosing private booths. Each of those areas have buttons that when pressed summon the waiter. As a teenager Mom dined there often, loving its atmosphere. Jill must have been impressed with me because we continued to date after that.

For some time she was my girlfriend and many guys in high school were jealous. They should have been. I lucked out finding this lovely classmate to break in the start of my high school years. We never got past first base, but it didn't matter.

Our last real date was towards the end of the second semester Freshman year. We dressed up and went to Old Orchard Country Club for dinner and a play. It was a four-course meal followed by the performance.

I wasn't old enough to drive and neither was she so Mom played chauffeur just this once. Jill's Mom came too. They had their dinners at the bar while Jill and I, pretending to be grown-ups on a school night, sat in the dining room looking like adults. The waitstaff treated us like a prince and princess which was a huge turning point in my life.

I craved living that way. Forever. Like a prince with a princess.

It was most exciting when our waiter asked if I wanted to review the wine list. Coloring my mustache with Mom's eyebrow pencil must have worked!

But alas! Nothing lasts forever. In June, as soon as school was out, Jill and her mom went on vacation. I didn't hear from her for 10 days and since cell phones had not yet been introduced, I had severe separation anxiety. When she returned from her "houseboat-cruise down the Mississippi" summer vacation she advised me we were sort of over.

No. We were over.

What to do? I spent a lot of time working on my art. Drawing, painting, creating, building card houses. Willy and I rode our ten-speeds. We explored Lake Forest, a very wealthy suburb on the lakefront, peeking at big old mansions through manicured hedges and imposing iron gates. We also went downtown to lie in the sun at the Oak Street beach. Neither one of us used sunscreen—just oil or Ban de Soile.

I had been a diabetic for six and a half years when Mom became active in the American Diabetes Association. Its mission is to prevent and cure diabetes and improve the lives of all people affected by this disease (not only the diabetic but the families, too). My enthusiasm for bike riding prompted Mom to organize the non-profit's first bike-a-thon fundraiser. Everyone had to ride in it. That meant me. So, I hit up the regulars at the bar of Eddie's Lounge as sponsors. I rode 90 miles in about 5 hours, then almost passed out. But I went to work that night to collect the money from my supporters. There was no time to feel bad.

Regular physical activity is especially important for diabetics. But too much exercise can result in low blood sugar and we may end up on the ground looking like actress Linda Blair in the horror film, *The Exorcist*. If alone, the result could be fatal.

Once aware of my strength, I decided to ride my Raleigh touring bicycle to Lake Geneva to see my cousins at their weekend/summer home. Ten-year-old Ray came with me. If I fell off my bike due to low blood sugar, he knew what to do. We left early in the morning before Mom could tell us we couldn't go. Halfway there, just when the flat landscape was rippling into a few low hills, my bicycle let out a startling noise. One of its tires went flat. I switched tires with Ray (both of our bikes had quick release hubs) and continued on my way. Ray phoned home from a gas station pay phone where he waited for Mom.

The following summer I tried to return to Lake Geneva on my own. Roaring down the highway on a motorcycle Dad bought us to ride around our backyard, I was stopped by a policeman as I crossed the Wisconsin State line. I was not wearing a helmet and Wisconsin has a helmet law. A good law if I do say so myself. The uniformed officer asked to see my driver's license.

"I don't have one."

"You mean you don't have one with you," Officer Friendly gave me the benefit of the doubt.

"No. I just don't have a license." I cannot tell a lie.

At some point during our short discussion, I admitted to being 15. He asked if I was running away from home. I told him NO, I had to be at work by five. It was Thursday and there was 300 pounds of fish waiting for me to bread.

What I regarded as an infraction he considered a crime against humanity. He made me leave my blue Harley Davidson on the side of the road, locked me in the back seat of his squad car, and drove to the Walworth County police station with the sirens blaring and the lights flashing. Someone there seized my belt and shoelaces before locking me in a cell. With my one phone call I phoned home.

This was a few years before *ET.*

Mom was at work. Dad was making sales calls. I asked Ray to cover for me at the restaurant which was his entre` to working at Eddie's. Soon a cop told me Mommy called. She informed him I was diabetic and demanded the officer give me something to eat. Jell-O. He gave me Jell-O.

I pictured my parents rushing to my rescue but to teach me a lesson they didn't show up for six or seven hours. It's not like I learned French or Spanish while incarcerated though I played poker through the bars with an older motorcycle guy and learned he had been there much longer than I. Apparently his Mommy or Daddy weren't coming. As soon as my family arrived, I was released from captivity. When Mom saw me without my belt or shoelaces she burst into tears, but Dad hailed a boys-will-be-boys smile. I think he was proud of me for getting caged. Sort of a rite of passage, but to please Mom he grounded me and sold the motorcycle.

I'd have to get a car.

And I did. Still not old enough to drive, the little old lady who sold me the Matador Red, 1964 Cadillac de Ville convertible with pointed fins and a white leather interior didn't ask to see my driver's license. I counted out $600.00 cash, put my bicycle in the trunk and drove home.

Beside the basics, Math, Science, English, Social Science, PE and Lunch, I signed up for Art. It was an elective class taught by Ilene Tandalaya Zuckerman. I loved her. She was a work of art with this gigantic mop of black hair and a warm, sexy smile.

I took art classes every semester of high school. In the second half of my freshman year I labored for weeks on a charcoal drawing entered in the Midwest Regional Scholastic Art competition. My crazy still life, drawn with white and black chalk on a bluish grayish paper, won first place. Ms. Zuckerman encouraged me to continue studying art.

Hooked, I joined Art Club. It met for an hour every day after school giving me just enough time to put away my supplies and bike to Eddie's Lounge. I was a star, and the commissions were coming in. Bob the Butcher, who drank at the bar every single night including Sundays, wanted pastoral murals on canvas for his shop. An uncle paid me to burn some images of ducks onto hides of suede with a wood burner. He had them framed and gave them to the president of Florsheim Shoes for his executive office.

Who would have thought years later my friend Shayle would buy the Florsheim building, convert it to lofts, and have my firm create the models, lobby and common areas? I lived there for 20 years, first in my Egyptian Temple and later in a penthouse with an enormous outdoor terrace. Afterwards, I moved to the other side of the river all the way east to Lake Shore Drive.

In Art Club, I met a new seductress. Leana. We were both aspiring artists and seemed to have a lot in common. She was popular with the boys and an upper-class person but despite that, we hit it off and spent a lot of time together working on our art.

At the same time, Willy dated a girl from Arlington Heights High School who worked at the movie theater. Jacqui, the candy counter / popcorn girl, wore CFM pumps to school and smoked in the Okay Corral on break. She did not have big boobs like Leana, but they both were juniors when Willy, Jacqui, Leana and I double dated.

Our idea of fun was collecting stemware from the finest hotels DOWNTOWN. We got dressed up in our Saturday night best and drove to the big city in my Caddy. I would drive down and Willy would drive back giving each couple plenty of make-out time in the big backseat. We brought a blanket for privacy, but once it blew away when the top was down.

In the city, we went from floor to floor at four and five-star hotels, on the prowl for stemware left on room service carts. Wine and water glasses. Champagne flutes. We each wanted a set of something. Made us feel well-heeled.

After several Saturdays, I ended up with service for eight from the Drake Hotel while Leana got a set from the Ambassador East (the hotel with the famed Pump Room). Willy's tulip-shaped glasses were from Arnie's, an authentic, uber gorgeous, art deco-styled palace with the city's most lavish Sunday brunch. We ate there for hours, always noticing another spectacular detail of the décor, returning to the various buffet tables for one more serving of eggs benedict and sausages and, of course, chocolate cake and cheesecake and carrot cake and pudding with whipped cream. It was so good, but awful for me. Awful because I ate all of it.

If I ate too much without taking enough insulin my blood sugar levels would rise along with the potential development of diabetic complications. This is what diabetics can expect if we don't take proper care of ourselves. Ultimately, I would deal with most of them due, in part (a big part), to my rebellious nature.

When Willy turned 20, we agreed he knew more than we did. And what did that include? Yes. You got it. DISCO.

THAT'S WHERE THE HAPPY PEOPLE GO

For the longest time, all we did was dream about going to discotheques. Willy introduced us to the music, and we LOVED it. If Jacqui, Leana, Willy and I weren't working at our assorted part time jobs, we were in my basement practicing our dance moves. One, two, three, one, two, three, step and… the Bump, the Swing and of course, the Bus Stop.

Enter cousin Judy.

She was Mom's first cousin who worked as a freelance photographer and advertising consultant. She also lived in Arlington Heights with her husband, a Spaniard, whom she met while studying abroad. How could Judy help us escape our ordinary suburban lives and find excitement in the big city?

Willy "acquired" his brother Edward's membership card to the BBC (Bombay Bicycle Club), a glamorous private disco where they filmed scenes from the movie *Looking for Mr. Goodbar* starring Richard Gere and Diane Keaton.

We wanted in.

Judy obliged by photographing the card and changing names (this was long before Photoshop, so talent was a must). Willy, Judy and I became preferred members.

As far as we knew it was *The Best Disco in Town.* At 16, I dressed in a black velvet suit, even in the summer, and carried a black lacquered, silver-tipped walking stick ala Fred Astaire. Leana was discofied to the nines, like Cinderella in her metallic sequin Quiana nylon dress with plunging neckline and platform shoes.

The four of us wore platforms. We were so very vogue way before Madonna.

Everyone dressed to kill or the bouncer, the illustrious Mr. T, wouldn't admit you even with a preferred membership card. His gold neck-chains and other jewelry came from the customers who lost them in the banquettes, on the dance floor, or at the assorted bars. Along with controlling violence, his job was to keep out the drug dealers and users. The disco scene included a flourishing recreational drug subculture. The right ones enhanced the experience of dancing to the deafening music and flashing lights. Disco-goers wanted cocaine and more. The movie *54* about Steve Rubell's world famous NYC discothèque tells the story best.

As innocent, certainly naive kids from the suburbs, we didn't know anything about that aspect of the disco scene. We just wanted to escape our humdrum suburban lives and pretend to be young sophisticates. Playing dress up expertly and with fake ID's, we drank lots of bizarrely named, sugary sweet, brightly themed cocktails of the disco era—the *Kamikaze, Long Island Ice-Tea, Harvey Wallbanger* and, when we were really feeling over 21, *Sex on the Beach.*

Sisters Sledge recorded a song about us. We were the greatest dancers. Practice in my basement paid off. When we stepped onto the backlit plexi dance floor everyone, and I do mean everyone, watched. On the balcony overlooking the dance floor members crowded the railing to study our every move although they would never admit it.

On school nights we closed the BBC around 2 am after dancing to songs like *Cher Chez la Femme* by Doctor Buzzard's Original Savannah Band or *Don't Take Away the Music* by Tavares and *Get Dancin* by Disco Tex and the Sex-O-Lettes. Throw in some dry ice smoke and we were in heaven even if it stung our eyes a bit. Those nights were our dreams come true until I took Leana home. She had to knock on her brother's bedroom window to get in. At 17 her parents always locked the doors and refused to give her a key. That was her home life.

At my home, we were crushed to learn Dad had a girlfriend. Night after night my uber Catholic mother criticized herself on the phone to her mother and sisters. She was angry. Depressed. And worried. Where did she do wrong? How could this happen to her?

There were signs of trouble for some time. Occasionally, when I came home from Eddie's Lounge, showered and changed into my pajamas, Mom asked me to get dressed. We'd drive past the girlfriend's house. If Father's car was parked in her driveway, Mom would lay on the horn, waking up the neighborhood. I never saw so many lights suddenly turn on at 11:30 pm. "Bad Daddy" as we so aptly called him, would come to the door and shake his fist at us.

"See that," she'd say, pointing, "I knew it".

Then we'd take off down the street. Tears flowed all the way home where she would throw herself down on their bed and cry the night away. Maybe take a Valium. Cindy said she was addicted to them back then, but I was clueless about that.

It was awful for the whole family. Worried about Mom we felt so wounded.

Being the oldest, I vowed to do something.

Our only phone was in the hallway outside the bedrooms. Sitting on the stairs leading to my lair with the door at the top of the stairway partially open, I could secretly hear Mother's conversations. That's how I learned Bad Daddy's girlfriend was a waitress at Henrici's Lobster and Steak House in Arlington Heights.

I had to meet her.

Of course, I couldn't go alone, so I reined in Leana, Willy and Jacqui. We cut school. By then we were pro's at it. Trying to look like adults… adults who could afford lobster and steak and drink wine served in a carafe at lunch time. We played dress up but probably looked more like theatre students. Again Mom's eyebrow pencil helped.

The restaurant had a gay '90's theme. Red damask wall-covering above dark oak paneling and a fake tin ceiling. Gaslight-style brass light fixtures dimly lit the interior. We approached the hostess stand as Jacqui, smoking her cigarette in a long glittery holder, requested we be seated with Barbara.

The hostess eyed us up and down undoubtedly wondering where we came from. Residents of Chicago's northwest suburbs did not play dress-up the way we did. We were hastily escorted to a table.

"Barbara will be with you shortly. Enjoy your luncheon."

Trying to guess which waitress was ours we looked around the room. Each wore deep V corsets that pushed their partially exposed breasts up to their noses, black seamed nylons, and CFM pumps. We made bets. Was it the one with the triple processed blonde hair so dry it would break if you ran your fingers through it? Or the redhead with several holes in her worn nylons? When Barbara came to our table, she was not what we expected. Not a beauty queen. Rather ordinary looking. More a plain Jane. Or is it Jayne?

She handed us red leather menus asking if we knew what we wanted to drink. I was going to order a Tab like a good diabetic. I was thirsty. Was my sugar high from the stress of the moment? Willy waved his hand to quiet me, telling Barbara we were celebrating and would like a bottle of champagne. She retrieved a wine list which he graciously accepted. We bit our lips to keep from laughing.

When Plain Jane returned, Willy ordered a bottle of Taittinger Champagne Brut Reserve. I was impressed. Mostly because I didn't know a thing about champagne except it had bubbles and made a noise when the cork was "popped."

A bus boy brought four champagne flutes. Barbara returned with the bottle and a stand. She opened it with great showgirlship. Willy sampled the subtle, pale gold beverage and approved.

Surprise!

He could have told her it tasted like vinegar, demanding she take it away. But he was sweet as pie. She poured the champagne, ladies first, without asking anyone for an ID.

"Would you like to order?"

We looked at each other, nodding. We were ready. Jacqui started with a half dozen oysters Rockefeller, then a Caesar salad with anchovies (yuck), and her main course, the surf and turf. She noticed they had Crème Brule which she ordered with the rest of her selections knowing how long it took to prepare. Not a fan of oysters, Leana started with the soup du jour—lobster bisque, a wedge salad with blue cheese, and a 2.5-pound lobster—she didn't want anything too big. Since they were all there to help me, I let Willy order next.

When we finished ordering, Plain Jane seemed happy. It was going to be a rather substantial bill for lunch, and she was already spending her anticipated tip.

The food was okay, not the legendary Pump Room quality we experienced on more than one occasion, but not mediocre. We were exceedingly nice to our waitress as I studied her during our encounter. With another bottle of Tat or was it two? And knowing how much we ordered, we left something from each course on our plates. Did not want to feel too stuffed.

Finally, we were done. Appetizers. Salads. Entrées. Desserts. And champagne. I asked for the check. Yes, it was three bottles of champagne for the four of us. Big wow. The bill was almost $800.00, for lunch, without the tip. Trying to hide my shock I looked at my guests. They nodded in agreement. I waved to Jane.

"Excuse me," I handed her the check in its leather cover. There was no credit card or cash accompanying it. "My father will pay for this…"

"Who is your father?" she asked unprepared for the shock of her life.

I told her.

Obviously, her teeth were real as they didn't fall out of her widely opened mouth. She stood frozen looking like the victim of a recent lobotomy.

"And you must know, none of us are old enough to drink. Could get you and this establishment into a lot of trouble…"

We left with her chin scraping the floor.

That night Dad called me from someplace unknown. He started yelling. Without listening to a word he sputtered, I hung up. I'd won a great battle, but the war was not over. Everyone in my house was affected by his betrayal and Mother's pain. I had done my best to give the old man a taste of his own medicine. On to the next mêlée!

Our parents quarreling sent Ray, Cindy and me looking for fun anywhere we could find it. It was easy to escape the constant madness of our *Little House NOT on the Prairie*. But Regina? She was only five. Teachers at her Montessori School taught her to play the violin but not how to meditate so she too could escape.

One Saturday night our house was uninhabited. Everyone fled the craziness of our little world leaving me home alone with Regina. My curious baby sister wanted to go to a disco. I told her so many stories about the clubs and she watched Willy, Jacqui, Leana and me practice in the basement. That night I asked if she wanted to go to one.

Leana and I were regulars at a club in a neighboring suburb. Disconnection also had a backlit Plexiglass dance floor, colored theater lights suspended from the ceiling and black walls. On certain nights, Paul Drake the DJ, broadcast his mixes on a local radio station.

The minute we walked through the door Regina was a celebrity. Everyone talked to her. She took the name of a song to the DJ booth and Paul played it immediately with a shout out to her. He was broadcasting. We had a drink. I behaved and ordered Tab. She had a Shirley Temple. I asked her if she wanted to dance. She did. We did. And before we knew it, we had to rush home before anyone, meaning Mom, discovered her gone. It was 11 pm. Way past her bedtime. But even Regina needed a little escape.

I hated to see Mom unhappy. Her face was a permanent shade of red. I knew what was coming, but when? One night, after feeling Mom's pain for so long, I nearly had a fist fight with Dad calling him an asshole and some four-letter words too. Ordering him out of the house, I told him to never return. To my surprise, he agreed. I was shocked. Mom was crying. Cindy was crying. Ray was crying. Regina clutched my leg wailing. She said she wanted to go back to the disco.

"What?" Mom didn't understand.

"Nothing," I replied trying to suppress my laugh. Like Sid Caesar told me, if you don't laugh, you're gonna cry.

A STAR IS BORN

Many of the situations I've faced have been the result of my choices, but that doesn't negate the fact the gods also handed me a platter full of obstacles. My choice has almost always been to make life amazing, no matter what. In my lifetime, I have done that over and over again.

In the same eighth grade where I was "removed" from the pro bono position of school newspaper editor, I played the lead in a production of the musical *You're a Good Man, Charlie Brown* and sang about my kite. It gave me a desire for show business I've never lost. I don't know if I was chosen because I had talent, or looked pathetic, or was the self-appointed director. It didn't matter.

Afterward, I threw a cast party in my basement. Some of the kids smuggled in liquor and guess what? They got drunk. My parents did not appreciate our youthful enthusiasm. Mom came down the stairs to investigate the screaming. Our cherry pie-eating contest became a pie-throwing slapstick extravaganza. Turning the last step, a pie flew past her face and hit the Z-Brick wall. The timing could not have been better; two more seconds and it would have hit her in the face. Cherry pie was all over the red brick veneer and black mortar. At least the color sort-of blended in. Well, not the crust.

I was grounded big time. On the spot.

"Two weeks," Mom declared.

Of course, I had only been drinking Tab. No beer or wine and certainly not liquor. I wasn't old enough. And I had no clue as to who really brought the alcoholic beverages. Well (long "L") maybe I did, but I wasn't a snitch.

My friends' and other kids' parents (a lot of people showed up) were called to retrieve their children. They were in no condition to ride their bicycles or even walk home. And the school principal, the one who relieved me of my job as editor of the school paper, came after class the following day to discuss my behavior. My folks were M-A-D. MAD!

I graduated from middle school in 1973 not knowing what I would be doing the rest of my life although throwing parties seemed like fun. But it was expensive—even when you asked everyone to bring something—like a cherry pie. So I needed a job. Delivering the newspaper for half a cent per copy was no way to pay for a party or two.

Having already read several inspirational books by W. Clement Stone including *Success Through A Positive Mental Attitude* and *The Success System That Never Fails,* I had an idea. During the dinner hour I went from one of our town's local bars to another shining shoes. I chose places where the commuters from downtown unwound after getting off their train from the city. They wore shoes they were eager to keep looking shiny and new.

I'd start at the beginning of a bar asking them, one by one, "Want a shine mister? Just a dollar…"

Most said yes and I always received a tip. At least another dollar. Often, I would get a five. In one hour, I could make $20.00 to $25.00 or more, amounting to $100.00 a week plus or minus, depending on how many days I chose to work. And I had no one to answer to. I was my own boss.

Just had to keep the customers happy.

When times were good, OR in the winter, I paid Ray to schlep my custom-made box of shoe waxes, brushes, and spray water from home to bar to bar to bar. It was a seven-block walk to the first one. He was ten.

I considered myself a capitalist because after meeting my expenses and payroll and giving Ray more money than he would have made delivering newspapers, I was able to buy for myself the bicycle, clothing, and whatever else Dad could not afford to purchase for me. After depositing money in my savings account, I still put cash in my pocket to visit the Yankee Doodle Dandy or Burger King. McDonalds (their fries and a Big Mac are still my favorite) was too far away to go with friends, unless the friend had a car. The dietician my pediatrician sent me to, did not approve of any of these fast-food delicacies. So, I didn't tell her.

THE SHOW
MUST GO ON

It was Cindy's 15th birthday. Seated around the dining table, my parents finally broke the news that was no news to us. They were divorcing. It was for the best they said.

"Who's best?" I wondered.

Mom excused herself and went to her bedroom. Through the closed door we could hear her crying. Dad got up from the table and left our house to go back to wherever. The four of us had cake.

"Make a wish," I said after we sang the happy birthday song. A little diversion and a moment of togetherness. Life.

Besides going to high school and washing dishes and breading fish at Eddie's Lounge, I sometimes worked backstage at the Arlington Park Theater. When the theatre wasn't black that is. Even though it was in the suburbs, the production of the plays equaled those in Chicago. I know because Mom took me to see *Tommy* and *Jesus Christ Superstar* when I was still just a kid. We sat in the nosebleed section close to God but I loved it nonetheless.

In Arlington Park Theatre, I organized the props making certain each accessory was ready when needed. My cohorts and I changed sets in seconds. When the stage went black between scenes, we'd run down the aisle, remove all the furniture and accessories on stage and replace them with an entirely new set. All in less than a minute. Sometimes one of us would fall causing the rest of us to trip over each other. It was very exciting.

One of our productions was a glamorous version of *Arsenic and Old Lace* with John Carradine, Eva Gabor of *Green Acres* fame, and her sister, Zsa Zsa Gabor, the "housekeeper". She always said she was a good housekeeper; when she got divorced (eight times) she kept the house. The sisters detested each other. Insisting on separate limousines from their downtown hotel they agreed on only one thing—Halston couture for their costumes.

Zsa Zsa was on her sixth husband, Jack Ryan, creator of Mattel's Barbie Doll. Jack had his own ideas for the play. One night he assumed the role of the dead body in the window seat with a dozen long stem red roses. When Zsa Zsa threw open the bench seat, John Carradine was supposed to pick up the dead body (me for months) and toss it into the cellar (orchestra pit). I always landed there with a big "Ugh!". That's when she told me I should be an actor.

This evening, Zsa Zsa was stunned to see her husband in my place. She slammed shut the lid of the bench seat and then opened it again enquiring, "Dahlink, vhat are you doing dare?"

The audience had no idea what transpired, but backstage we were having the time of our lives. After weeks and months of the same line after line, we enjoyed the switch. So did Zsa Zsa and her husband.

During *Double Take,* starring Sid Caesar and Imogene Coca, I was certain my life in the professional theater was over. In a scene of the Neil Simon play, Sid faints. Dressed completely in black (so no one would see me), I was supposed to hand Imogene smelling salts. By mistake, I gave her a chicken leg! When the play was over, she hurried backstage to ask who handed her the dark meat. Raising my hand, I stepped forward. She rushed over and gave me a big hug, thanking me for mixing things up.

The legendary Hollywood movie stars I worked with were unexpectedly considerate of me. Fetching a glass of whole milk for Leslie Caron before every show was not work, it was an honor. She always said thank you and was very appreciative. One evening, as I held the door for Zsa Zsa who was getting ready to walk on stage, she stopped for a second and told me how handsome I looked. I was a geeky 16-year-old wearing a plaid leisure suit over a light blue sweater. It was so 70's. But I never forgot that moment.

It was in the theatre that the professional use of my creativity was ignited. Exposed to the art of creating illusions using fabrics, furniture, and damn good lighting I loved working there. But the theatre went bankrupt after each production and was ultimately converted into an awesome disco. *Cinderella Rockefeller.*

My theater life greatly influenced my design career. John Robert Wiltgen Design, Inc. is renowned for creating exceptionally "dramatic" award-winning homes.

Somewhere near the end of my sophomore year Willy asked me to work at the paint store. He said Mrs. Donahue knew me to be hard working, dependable and pleasant. I was her first choice for the position.

When I gave my two weeks' notice at Eddie's Lounge, Mrs. Jensen, the owner, was sad. She said I was the best dishwasher, fish breader, bar stocker EVER. As such, she gave me a going away party complete with a buffet supper including homemade chocolate cream pie (my favorite) and told me to invite whomever I wanted.

During the merrymaking, Leana and I danced to *Zing Went the Strings of My Heart*, the disco version by The Tramps, wowing the drunken patrons with our moves. When I tried to dip Leana but threw her onto the dirty floor the customers applauded enthusiastically.

At my new job Willy taught me how to mix custom paint colors for customers, often matching a color in the wallpaper they just bought from us. Sometimes, on our day off, he and I installed the wallpaper too. Anything to make a buck! Both of us needed the money. At 16 and 20 we were working our way down Chicago Magazine's list of better restaurants.

With our busy work schedules, Leana and I cut school regularly to do homework. My good penmanship enabled me to write notes, ostensibly from Mom, claiming another diabetic catastrophe. I signed her name adding her business phone number beneath it. That always worked. Leana would call the principal's office speaking in her parents broken Macedonian accent, which nobody understood.

We would either go to my house to practice our dance moves or drive downtown for fresh strawberries with cream at the newly opened Ritz-Carlton Hotel hidden inside the marble-clad

Water Tower Place. We were impressed when white gloved doormen opened the doors for us. It wasn't a true break from school because after breakfast at The Café, we studied in The Terrace, opposite the hotel's bigger than life marble and bronze fountain featuring a group of cranes with their wings spread. For two kids from the middle of suburban nowhere, we discovered a splendid study hall.

After work, Leana and I went out dancing. We won numerous dance contests. The Hustle. The Swing. Even the freestyle. Some contests had cash prizes. Other a substantial bar tab. Often, we didn't start until after Arlington Heights' curfew. Her mother would chase my car with broom in hand as we backed out of the driveway. I crept away ever so slowly just to let her think she might catch us. I know she hated me, but we just wanted to have fun. In our minds, we were doing nothing wrong. And, like most teenagers, we were always right!

New Year's Eve, I invited Leana to the theater for our latest production, *Brief Lives,* a British play about a 17th-century Englishman who met and kept accounts of many of the famous men of his day. It became one of the most successful one person shows in history. The famous British actor, Roy Dotrice, starred. It was a big deal. I was supposed to pick her up at 7:00 pm for the 7:30 curtain. Then we would go to dinner at the Top of the (adjacent) Hilton. Except Willy and Jacqui had other plans for me.

Wanting to fix me up with another girl from our school who also drove a red Cadillac convertible, they abducted me. Jacqui hoped she and I, and our cars, would become quite the couple. Jacqui and Leana were either best friends or they hated each other. They were always competing. Who was prettier? Who was the better dancer? Who was more in love? This was one of those times when the two weren't getting along. I couldn't call Leana to cancel as there were no cell phones yet. I just didn't show up at the arranged time.

She was dressed, I am certain, looking more beautiful than ever and waited and waited and waited. She called my house multiple times. No one knew what to say. In the meantime, I was downtown with two of my best friends and Allison, a girl I never met before. Along with a million others, we went to State Street for the countdown. It was mayhem and I hated it.

I phoned Leana the next day not quite sure what to say. She made it easy hanging up on every call. Why didn't I resist Willy and Jacqui? They knew I had plans. I wasn't interested in meeting this Allison girl. Even if she drove a red Cadillac convertible that was newer than mine. But mine was nicer; it had fins! Leana didn't speak to me for months.

Who could blame her?

During the Leana-less second semester of my junior year, I attended Winter Ball with my friend Pam. She was voted the one most likely to marry a millionaire. And she did. Twice. Her first husband, Clement Stone (son of the man who's books I read back in 8th grade) was 30 years older than her and had a heart attack the night of their wedding. Five or six weeks before the big do he presented her with a pre-nup which she refused to sign. Pam ordered him to call their 500 guests and tell them the wedding was off. Clem did not want to be socially embarrassed and so the wedding went on as planned. That night he was rushed to the hospital where he died 3 months later.

Pam inherited a 22,000 square foot David Adler manse in Lake Forest. A home in Acapulco. And a full floor co-op downtown where she met her second husband. Dirk Lohan was 21 years older, the grandson of Mies Van der Rohe and had a better heart than Clem. I ended up with clients who were presumably millionaires including one of Pam's stepsons.

Yep. It's a small world after all.

Leana and I were still in the same art class. We planned it that way when we made our class selections the previous semester. Eventually she had to speak to me. We were meant to be together.

Then something amazing happened. She won a full, four-year art scholarship to Arizona State University. Even though it was announced over the school PA system not many of her classmates understood how much this meant to her. Her parents did not support her interest in art or anything else. In 1976, the women's lib movement was in the public eye every day, yet her folks believed she should live at home, with them (God forbid), until she got married. Her uncle Boris lived with his mother until the day she died (which was in her 80's). He never got married. So Leana broke down and told me she was getting out, providing the chance I needed to make a real apology. I congratulated her on this awesome opportunity. It was the only way she could go to college, and I was proud of her. She was so brave.

A few days later she was to appear on *the Ray Rayner Show*, a children's television program of the 1960's and 70's, to talk about her art and scholarship. Her parents would not drive her to the TV station even though our school approved the day off. Of course, I volunteered. After her 7:00 am appearance, we ended up at the Ritz to celebrate over breakfast. I was so happy things were back to normal.

The school year was ending. Leana was graduating. Seniors finished classes two weeks earlier than the rest of the student body. What was I going to do at Arlington High School without her? I was so distraught I didn't go to school either. Instead, I spent the time off with her. My reason for absence? Cindy, a freshman, told all my teachers I had mono.

Though Leana worked extra hours at Carol's Casuals, a dress shop, to earn as much money as possible before leaving for college, there was not a day when we didn't see each other. We always made time for holding each other as we danced the night away. Sundays, if the weather was nice, Willy, Jacqui, Leana and I went to Oak Street beach to people watch and work on our tan lines. I drove. We all loved riding in the red Cadillac convertible with the top down.

Before we knew it, summer was over and it was time for her to leave.

I felt awful watching her mother shake Leana's hand goodbye. There were no hugs. No kisses. No emotions. No love. Leana packed everything that ever meant anything to her into the two suitcases she was allowed on the plane.

Willy, Jacqui, and I drove her to O'Hare Airport. In those days, anyone, not just passengers could walk to the gate. After we were done hugging and kissing, the three of us watched her board the plane. She was the last passenger on, and we waited until the attendant secured the door to the jet bridge.

My friends thought I needed a Dairy Queen to cheer me up. Like that would help. It didn't but I found it hard to say no to a chocolate ice cream cone dipped in chocolate. Afterward, I dropped Willy and Jacqui off at her house and went home. I couldn't believe Leana was gone. How could it be? Throwing myself on my twin bed I cried.

For days.

HELP ME

One sunny August afternoon, still dealing with my retinopathy I convinced myself my vision cleared sufficiently
to drive. I could see better than when I chauffeured Cynthia to
and from NYC. The sun was shining in my eyes as I headed
west. Maybe a good pair of Persol sunglasses could cure the
whole debacle.

Driving on a busy expressway to a client's home in prestigious
Barrington Hills, my good eye suddenly started bleeding. Like
an out-of-control lava lamp, I began to see the blood swirling
behind it. Within minutes I lost all my vision. I maneuvered
my white Ford Granada onto the gravel shoulder, put on the
flashers, took a deep breath, and waited for help. I did not have
a cell phone; it was 1983, they were brand new at the time and
far too expensive. Sightless, I could not walk along the side of
the highway.

I sat there struggling to see the speeding cars. Thankfully,
my car's battery didn't die before help came.

Eventually, I heard someone pull off the road behind me. A
car door opened and closed. Gravel crunched beneath heavy

footsteps. The good Samaritan approached asking if I needed help. I must have looked perfectly fine to him wearing my pristine light gray suit and GQ tie.

I explained the situation as efficiently as possible trying not to give into panic. He did not have a cell phone either but promised to use the next exit to call my home from a pay phone. I thanked him profusely.

I couldn't see the clock on the dashboard. I had no sense of time. I just listened to the cars whizzing past. Eventually Mom and Dad found me. I didn't need sight to know she had been crying. I visualized streaks of mascara running down the round cheeks of her Polish face.

"What were you thinking?" she asked sympathetically as she climbed in on the driver's side.

"I had an appointment with a client. I am trying to run a business…" I refused to think about it anymore. To forget my predicament, I fell asleep. I was shutting down.

By the time Mom's foot hit the gas pedal to merge into traffic, I was out.

At home, she sat me down at the dining table.

"John, we have something to talk to you about…"

I didn't say anything.

"We've sold the house…"

Oh my God.

"…and are moving to Texas!"

"What?"

"You can come with us."

Over my dead body.

"There will always be room for you…"

And rattle snakes.

"...But we are leaving next week."

"I have a job down there," that was my father. He finally spoke up. "so, we have to git going real soon..."

Dad was already talking like a Texan. He was such a phony. Why couldn't Mom see that? I don't know how she could have married him. Again.

"...but you don't have to be out of the house for three more months."

Ray would be here for most of the summer, until he left for college. After high school he took a gap year and worked his buns off to save money for his education. Now he was ready to leave, ironically, for Texas A & M. Didn't matter. I would take care of myself if only I could see the calibration on my syringes.

"John how are you going to survive?" Mom was worried. That's what Mother's do.

Guess what? I was worried, too.

I couldn't see. I had a mortgage on a building that John and I started tearing apart. I had a business with an office and clients and products on order. Some of those deliveries could take four to six months. Even if I wanted to go with them, which I didn't, I could not just "git up and go" as my father said. I had responsibilities. If I wanted to succeed, I had to act like an adult. In fact, I was an adult. I was 22.

Dr. Fetkenhour said it could take a month or more for the blood to be absorbed in the back of my eyes after the bleed. Until then, I couldn't see enough to survive on my own. I needed help.

Susan Wachholz, Leana's friend from ASU and Cynthia Rowley's Chicago roommate was my choice. No. Make that my salvation. She was very style conscious. As a photography major, she had a discriminating eye and, for some reason, was a wiz at bookkeeping. So, when I learned my family was leaving, that they sold our house, I surprised Susan by offering her half of John Robert Wiltgen Design, Inc. I couldn't stay in business without someone competent and stylish. There simply was no one else like her that I knew. Well, Cynthia. But she was busy doing her own thing which has paid off immensely.

Susan was an inspiration and supremely loyal. We were simpatico because we both longed for life in the faster lane.

When my family arrived in Texas, it turned out my father didn't have a job. He lied. Didn't he know we would find out? Fortunately, Mom's company, Hertz Rent-A-Car, transferred her to their Houston office. They valued her work ethic.

Having a hard time seeing and no place else to go, I finally moved in with Grandma and Grandpa Niemec when Ray left for school. Work slowly progressed on the Bucktown three-flat as John and I were both working full-time to make money. My grandparents' home was closer to Chicago, so it wasn't as far for Sue to drive every day. She picked me up each morning. Park Ridge was fourteen miles from downtown Chicago which, during rush hour, was an hour's drive for her each way. At the end of the day, she returned me to my grandparents. She always walked me to the door to make sure I didn't trip on the concrete step. Often, she would come in and talk to Grandma and Grandpa. Unlike Dolly Parton she was not working 9 to 5, but she never complained.

Sometimes I volunteered to take the train to Park Ridge in the evening. When exiting the train, I would ask a fellow passenger to turn me in the direction of a waiting cab. Arriving at my grandparents, I would open my wallet instructing the driver to take the money he needed. Once that proved not the smartest idea. Not everyone was as honest as I expected. After being ripped off, Sue put assorted amounts of money in different pockets, so I could take out ten dollars and ask for change.

I had so many things to learn!

At work, the men's room was down the hall from our office. In the beginning, getting there was a task. I wouldn't let Sue help. Instead, when I had to go, she called the elderly janitor who walked me into the men's room and positioned me in front of a urinal.

"If you aim straight ahead, you'll do just fine," he said and walked away.

Eventually, by counting footsteps and feeling my way past the stalls to the urinals, I found my own way. And *yes*, I always washed my hands.

Sue was my eyes for so many things. When I couldn't see at all, she ran to the Merchandise Mart to scout furniture for our design jobs. She selected items she wanted me to see—well, feel actually—before we showed them to a client. Salespeople stared when I walked into a glass wall dividing the to-the-trade showrooms from the reverently silent corridors. That happened so many times I was certain I would eventually need a nose job. Finally, Sue would take my arm and lead me to the intended piece where I would get down on my hands and knees to feel the furniture.

"What is this little thing here?" I might ask quietly.

"That is the way they upholstered the ottoman. It is shirred and there is a fabric-covered button in the middle." She sounded like a pro even though she had no design training.

The salespeople learned what was happening and tried to help. If Sue called ahead, the showroom staff cleared a path to prevent me from falling over a coffee table.

I might have chosen a career more suitable to my circumstances.

Grandma Niemec was impressed with the way I did my own laundry and ironed my button-down shirts for work when I couldn't see. Lying on her sofa in the family room munching chocolate candy, watching the new nighttime soap opera, *Dynasty*, she assured me I could always open a Chinese laundry if the design thing didn't work out.

CAN YOU SEE
ME NOW?

A year later, the 3-flat progressed to a point where I was able to move in. Ray was home for the summer making more money to stay in college, so he moved in too. A new roof kept us from getting soaked. New windows let the sunshine in and kept the bugs out. The electrical and drywall work was complete. We had a new kitchen and bath, but the rest of our place was still a work in progress.

Sue and I were busy designing our little world and I had been quite lucky. Dr. Fetkenhour's laser art seemed to be working. He stopped the growth of new blood vessels, cauterized the leaky ones and the fluid in the back of my eye was somewhat clear.

Then, in July I woke up one morning and it was as if someone turned on that fucking lava lamp again. I rolled my eyes to the right; I could see the blood rushing to that side. Then to the left, the blood stirred in that direction. Hysterical, I called Fetkenhour's office alerting them I was on my way.

Checking in with the receptionist, I desperately recited a few new Helen Keller jokes. I tried so hard to hide my fear and anger and frustration. She laughed with great understanding.

Fetkenhour examined both eyes but didn't say much. When Brigit turned the light back on, she sighed. He let out a deep breath. They sounded so ominous. New blood vessels broke. He wanted to try something different and said if I could wait, they would prepare another room for the procedure.

In the ultra-sterile chamber, he calmly explained death could occur from a retrobulbar injection. It never happened on his table but if the needle inadvertently punctured the optic nerve, anesthesia could travel to the brainstem. My hand shook signing the consent form. Brigit inserted an IV for sedation. They performed the procedure without any complications.

Fetkenhour's report concluded "The patient left the room in good condition," meaning I was still alive.

It took a long time for the blood to re-absorb before I could see well enough to read with thick magnifying glasses. I hated the impact this made on my freedom but kept reminding myself "You never know what worse luck your bad luck saved you from."

I experienced continuous problems with the vision in my left eye which leaked again requiring additional laser work. The sight was reduced to 20/80 meaning what a normal person saw from 80 feet, I had to move 60 feet closer to see.

I repeatedly told myself: I can handle this. I can handle this. But in February, I began seeing black spots in my *right* eye every morning. It was torture to realize my vision was slowly disappearing. Again. Before long problems in both eyes shrank my vision to 20/200.

I was legally blind.

Work was not only my passion, but my greatest distraction. Fortunate to have my own business; it kept my mind off the bigger problem. The legally blind diabetic one. Even though I could not see the patterns or textures of materials we were recommending, I worked by creating pictures in my brain of what I felt worked best in my clients' homes. I would not let them down.

Slowly, my left eye began clearing. Its overall vision improved to 20/70. Sue and I didn't dare tell my clients. After all, who would hire a blind interior designer?

One day my vision cleared enough for me to go it alone. I wanted to visit the new Holly Hunt showroom in the Merchandise Mart. I needed fabrics for a project. The striking showroom featured the most prestigious vendors. There my blood sugar bottomed out. As I stood near an Hermes leather sofa I began to stutter and wobble. A department manager noticed my hands and arms flailing uncontrollably. She didn't know what was happening. Was I drunk or on drugs? She telephoned Sue who told her to call 911.

Wearing a pair of black patent-leather Valentino shoes, Sue rushed to the scene. So did the paramedics. They found me thrashing about on the designer sofa. One medic held me down while another stuck me with an IV. I know he had trouble inserting the catheter because I bled all over the sofa which had a $22,000.00 price tag in 1984. The medics strapped me to the gurney, tore down the hall into an elevator. Sue tried keeping up while clutching my brief case, her bag, and tissues to wipe her tears.

Sitting in the front seat of the ambulance, between the driver and his assistant, the sirens were blaring. The driver looked at Sue, who was still crying, and said "those are really *hot* nylons you're wearing…" Not knowing what else to do she hit him repeatedly with her purse and my briefcase.

When it was safe for me to return to the Mart, the sofa was gone.

***

I accepted the request to design the master bath in a 40,000 square foot designer showcase house hoping it would buy me some publicity. My talents were being presented along with 29 other designers. Some far more seasoned than I. So, the publicity was not guaranteed.

Old and worn (the house, not me), it was the largest I'd ever been in. The master bath had potential and I was thrilled with my latest distraction. I commissioned a large art deco-style painting to unify a pair of "his" and "her tubs. They were side-by-side, and the artwork spanned the width of both creating an architectural relationship. Silk draperies framed a spectacular view. The bathroom was featured in numerous papers and magazines. "Bathrooms to die for" became a John Robert Wiltgen Design specialty.

My vision kept see-sawing between improving and getting worse. In June, I was hospitalized again. By this time, I stopped telling Mom. I was tired of her rushing from Texas so she could stand at the foot of my already uncomfortable hospital bed and cry. Or tell me people at their Texas church were praying for me. Grandpa's church folks in Tomahawk were praying for me too. Everyone was praying for me WHICH I HATED. It is so hard to believe in God when, at 23, the whole world needs to pray for you.

I hoped someone, other than God, was going to be able to help me. But I also prayed just to be safe.

During surgery, Fetkenhour brought a microscope into position for a *conjunctival peritomy*. This is not as much fun as it sounds. I'll spare the gory details. Like the part where he removed a strip of flesh from inside my eyelid OR placed a super cold metal probe against the back wall of the eye to cause ice formation within small blood vessels. I had three different surgeries in one week that were more like something from *Texas Chain Saw Massacre V.* Each operation addressed a different problem. I was angry. Depressed. Frightened. And running out of hope.

One morning, while finishing my diabetic breakfast of dry, cold scrambled eggs, two pieces of toast (also cold), a tab of frozen butter and a not too ripe banana, I sensed someone entering my hospital room. Both eyes were bandaged, but I heard light footsteps on the hard vinyl floor. Then another sound. Perhaps a vase being placed on the table next to my bed.

"Hello?" was it a nurse?

Two arms embraced me in a tight, long hug. Instinctively, the fragrance and size said Rhonda. Only Sue knew I was there, and she wouldn't call Rhonda. She wouldn't even call my mother.

Three years later Rhonda finally came clean to me...

"While we were together," she started. "I was an alcoholic and drug addict. I drank way too much and did coke. Not the sugar free kind you drink."

How else could she work all day and dance all night?

"It was hard to keep up with you!" she exclaimed.

"After our series of unfortunate incidents, I went to rehab, then AA and most recently the Unity Church. The church provides a lifestyle leading to health, prosperity, happiness and peace of mind."

Rhonda apologized for not revealing her problems earlier. She told me not to worry, I would get better. And that was it.

She was gone.

Was I hallucinating from the anesthetic?

Following my release there was a slight improvement in my right eye. I was thrilled. Perhaps Dream Rhonda was right.

Amid all this eye problem bullshit my office received a phone call from a very successful real estate developer and restaurateur inquiring about the possibility of our designing his vintage home built in 1895. After hearing the description of the 7,850-square foot mansion with separate coach house, I was eager to see the place. So I unwrapped the bandages myself and carefully cleaned around the eyes. Tried a little concealer. The natural me would make a much better impression than appearing before these potential clients looking like a version of the Boris Karloff Mummy. I didn't want to give them any reason for not hiring us.

When Sue picked me up the following morning, she screeched.

"That bad?" I asked.

"Does it hurt?"

"No, not really. I'm sure it looks worse than it is."

My eyes looked monstrous. No white part was visible, and the surrounding skin was black and blue as if I lost a back alley fight. What would the new client think?

We found out that evening when Sue pulled my car into the client's driveway.

"This is the most amazing house you have ever been asked to design. I wish you could see it!" She took my arm. "One step up, two, three, four, five, six, seven, eight," she whispered.

We didn't need to ring the bell of the imposing red granite Roman Revival structure. Bill Dec waited at the door. He was a big guy, a really, big guy. I could tell when we shook hands. I squeezed firmly.

"Wow," he was taken back. Not by the handshake. "What happened to your eyes?"

"Hay fever," I replied. "I have allergies."

"You too?" he asked.

I nodded.

"Yeah, my kids have hay fever. Let me tell Celia you are here." Ushering us in he led the way to the dining room where floor plans were spread on the table. Arm in arm, Sue and I followed. He introduced us to his wife, a petite Filipino woman. Then he walked us through their residence via the blueprints spread across their dining room table.

Sue sat next to me. That was our thing. Later she told me the dining room had remarkable moldings, pocket doors, and Adam-style pediments above cased openings. She did most of the talking because why? She was the one who could see. I suggested we walk through the house instead of trying to get inspired by blueprints.

"Great idea," said Bill. "I can tell you've done this before."

Bill and Celia led the way. Once again, Sue clutched my arm. "This is going to be tricky. Hold on tight."

The house had four floors but no elevator. I imagined it perfect for entertaining. The main floor featured a gracious gallery with a stately hand-carved staircase. On the right were the living room, dining room, and large kitchen with breakfast room. There was a two-story family room that someone added at the rear. The lower level was dark and creepy; Sue's first and lasting impression. It said deluxe wine and cheese cellar party room to me. There were five bedrooms. The master suite featured a fireplace, private outdoor terrace, separate dressing room and vintage bath. The children's bedrooms were scattered throughout the second and third floors. The attic included a large sitting room which became a home office.

It was 11:00 pm when we finished our interview. As Bill led us to the front door he said, "Send us your agreement. I can tell you two have a good *feeling* for old houses."

He didn't know how true that was.

A week later, I was back in Fetkenhour's office. The vision in my left eye was non-existent at 20/300. My right eye was hemorrhaging again. I could barely see shadows. And then, things got worse.

I was a mess—so sick and tired of this bullshit. How much more could I endure? Mom wanted me to move to Texas. The Lone Star State had excellent programs for the visually impaired, but how about some words of encouragement? Like… "Don't worry, honey. You're going to be fine."

Why couldn't she get it through her head I didn't want to be blind?

By mid-July my left eye allowed me to see obscurities and my right eye struggled to improve. At one point it recovered to

20/70. But by August, things worsened, and I needed more help getting around.

An ultrasound showed blood collecting behind the eye. I was legally blind. Again and again and again. My ability to see light diminished.

What was I going to do?

By the end of August my vision was 20/400 in both eyes. I had to let Sue and Steve, my assistant who prepared a lot of our drawings, do all their work and much of mine. I felt worthless and so depressed I intentionally skipped my next appointment with Fetkenhour.

What else could he do?

I fell down a rabbit hole and doubted I would ever be able to climb back out. The only logical explanation was I must have been a real asshole in one of my past lives!

Despite it all, I would not be deterred from seeing, well at least hearing, Sue exchange vows with Tom, her groom in a September ceremony. Even though I couldn't see much, the wedding seemed beautiful. Sue's floral arrangement was a copy of Princess Di's. Her dress had a long train. She and her new husband rode from the church to the Drake Hotel in a horse drawn carriage. During dinner, Franz Benteler strolled amongst the tables playing his Stradivarius violin. My date, a refined girl who never knew exactly what I could see, graciously offered to cut my chicken cordon bleu. Not wanting help, even hers, I diplomatically declined. Then immediately dropped a forkful all over my white linen jacket.

In November of 1984 I returned to the hospital for a totally unrelated problem. Severe pain in my right thigh was so bad it prevented me from walking. My right retina continued to bleed, not that it mattered. I couldn't see anyway. Dr. Fetkenhour said there was nothing he could do about my eye. I had to be patient and wait out the problem. It might improve. But the hospital pursued my leg problem. A new doctor for me, Claire Giegerich, an orthopedic surgeon, said I had cellulitis and put me on IV antibiotics.

Diabetics are at high risk of developing this bacterial skin infection. It occurs in areas that may have been damaged or are inflamed. Bad circulation from peripheral artery disease is also an unexceptional cause. Aside from local symptoms, it can also be accompanied by chills and fever, muscle aches, nausea and vomiting. This was my beginning of a long and debilitating 20-year battle.

WORKIN' DAY
AND NIGHT

In January of 1984, I officially moved John Robert Wiltgen Design, Inc. to the fourth floor "penthouse" level of our Bucktown building.

Penthouse. Smokehouse. Same thing. The rooftop office featured picture windows with south and west exposures and countless recessed lights which, later, enabled me to work around the clock, seven days a week.

John and I received rent from the tenants on the lower two floors and JRWD paid it's share for the penthouse. Plus, we had coin-op laundry equipment in the basement. By the time we added up our receipts, paid the mortgage and taxes, we made money living there.

My right eye improved remarkably, to 20/25. Although I was grateful, I did not allow myself to become elated over the change because I knew it was temporary. I was being realistic not negative. In February, Dr. Fetkenhour discovered a tiny split in my left retina. He said it needed careful observation. By the end of the month, hemorrhaging caused a sudden loss of vision in that eye. There was also a cruel change in the right eye.

I had to persevere.

Sue and I scheduled a meeting with the vice-president of a real estate firm that converted vintage rental apartment buildings into landmarked condominiums selling individual units to investors who bought them with an eight-year property tax freeze. We were to meet Susan Baldwin at one of three buildings.

We decided not to alarm the VP with my blindness. Having a lot of experience at not being able to see we perfected our act and expected to nail this prospect. The buildings were "works in progress" undergoing extensive renovation meaning piles of fallen rubble, holes in concrete floors, and other assorted dangers for anyone—not just someone who couldn't see.

"This is going to be another one of those tricky performances," my Sue whispered, laughing… the necessary absurdity. Walking arm in arm she attempted to prevent me from stumbling on debris in our path. After an hour or so of my "seeing" by being pulled this way and that, tripping over bricks, walking into walls and listening to both Sue's descriptive comments on the architecture and vintage charm, we proceeded to the second and third buildings for more of the same.

When finished, we chose a nearby faux-French brasserie for lunch. I followed the two blondes, grasping the back of my Sue's coat belt.

I thought I succeeded in pretending to "see" until, during our luncheon, the new Susan stopped in mid-conversation, observing "John, you have your menu upside down."

My Sue laughed dodging the bullet with a comment to me, "You are so good."

Turning to the new Susan she said, "John was just waiting to see how long it would take for you to notice. He tests our prospective clients to determine how observant they are. You passed." We made a deal with her firm to create the models and lobbies of three buildings as well as their corporate offices.

Zsa Zsa was right. I could have been a professional actor. I feel I am performing every day of my life.

Business was escalating even as my vision became blurrier and yellowed with the maturation of a cataract in my right eye. A different doctor, not Fetkenhour, was waiting until the cataract "ripened," as if being grown in a tomato patch. Today cataracts do not need to mature before they can be extracted. Modern advances in this surgery allow them to be removed at any stage of their development and a replacement lens inserted.

DO YOU WANT
TO DANCE?

In November of 1984, the lack of vision in both eyes prevented me from driving. I wanted to go out and listen to loud music so I couldn't hear myself think. It was either that or stay at home and slit my wrists.

I didn't know how much more I could take but the loud music wasn't as messy.

There still was no Uber and I didn't want to use a cab. I called my friend, Paul, a psychic, to find out what he was doing. Did he want to go out and could he come get me? It was 10:00 pm. He said he knew I was going to call and was happy to oblige. An hour later we were cruising in his vintage Cadillac with bigger fins than my first car. Great minds think alike!

He took me to a bar in the suburbs. Cheap drinks. Free parking. What did I care? I couldn't see so it didn't matter. He asked if I wanted to dance. *Let's Hear it For the Boy* the first big hit for Denice Williams was playing. Afraid of bumping into someone or stumbling off the elevated dance floor I declined and leaned up against a nearby post.

I enjoyed the music and heavy bass which drowned out all the thoughts in my head. A parade of cheap colognes passed by when along came a *parfum*. Its lingering scent was spicy.

Opium.

"You are the coolest guy here..." it was either a sexy female or fantastic drag queen. I wasn't quite sure and wondered who the person was addressing. I strained to hear more.

"Oh, so you're a snob," she shouted at the top of her lungs. "Sorry I bothered you."

"Were you speaking to me?" I shouted back.

"Yes." She sounded a bit farther away.

"I'm sorry. I can't see. I wasn't sure." I moved towards the voice.

"What do you mean you can't see? You're blind? Love your overcoat." I chose to stay warm in a black and brown tweed Armani overcoat I recently purchased on Oak Street while shopping with Gertrude. Another way I avoided depression. Unfortunately, one my insurance company did not reimburse me for.

We tried talking above the music. She was with friends and asked if I'd like to meet them?

"Sure."

She led me to a table away from the crowd. Her name was Athena, like the Greek virgin goddess.

Jeff was a friend of hers. Once introduced, he talked, and I listened. For a long time. He recently broke up with his manfriend of seven years, a car salesman. Not Jeff. The manfriend who is a Leo.

"I'm a Leo," I declared.

"You're a Leo? That's good. I get along with Leo's. I'm a Pisces...."

Really, I am not into all that astrology stuff. I'll listen and be amazed if something seems genuinely authentic, but so much of it is generalizations. Don't you think?

Jeff was living at home with his parents where he kept his three-foot Chinese Water Dragon in a cage. He went to the pet store weekly to buy live blind mice. His dragon liked them fresh.

"My mom is overprotective and worries about everything. When I was younger, she wouldn't let me cross the street and we lived on a dead-end. I was a manager at Flipside, a record store, and just started a new career as a hairdresser in a trendy suburban salon named Luigi and Salvo. Have you heard of it? I liked Grace Jones and was given the opportunity to pick her up at the airport and drive her around for two days while she performed at the Park West (a Chicago Club). I got the gig after sending her manager several portraits I painted of her. She's a bitch in real life. Absolutely destroyed my admiration of her. Hired as a driver, I told her manager I would use my parents' Cadillac but when the time came, I had to resort to my orange Gremlin. She was so contorted in the back seat she stuck her legs out the window. It was hilarious. She stayed at a Holiday Inn in Chicago's near west side skid row. It was gross. I couldn't believe she would stay there. While waiting in the hallway for her, I kept knocking on the door to warn her she would be late.

"Let them wait," Grace screeched back.

"When we finally got there, I was able to watch the show with the other stagehands. That was cool." Then, "My sister didn't finish high school. She has a son which makes me an uncle.

Me and my sister went to Catholic schools. In high school I was very fat and frequently beaten up on the bus. So, I lost a bunch of weight. Ever since then I watch what I eat. I love to dance. Do you want to dance?"

I said I loved to dance too, but no. Thank you. Maybe another time. I needed to find Paul who I'm sure was looking for me. He was my ride home. I told the group Paul resembled Fidel Castro and they found that guy right away. Jeff scribbled his phone number on a cocktail napkin. I gave him mine and left.

The next day, while Sue and I were working in the penthouse, the phone rang. It was Jeff. I could tell he was going to start rambling again, so I cut him off. But before I did, he asked if we could get together. He knew I couldn't drive so he agreed to come downtown even though he never drove in the city before.

He came over Friday night. My Grandma Wiltgen visited during the week and made me several meals, so we enjoyed a delicious dinner at the dining room table. When I was in Texas visiting Mom and Regina, we went to an auction house for the fun of it. I ended up with a hilarious Regency dining table with two columns for legs at each of the four clipped corners and an equally hilarious ball and claw foot recamier. They were my first authentic antique pieces and I treasured owning them for a long time. No joke!

My home was sparsely furnished. I was still spending money on completing the construction, but in 1984 the large open living/dining room and small bedrooms were carpeted in gray. That was way before the current trend which has been in vogue since the year 2000. I had a beautiful sectional covered in a fine green wool flanked by Regency tray tables. The dining room wall was mirrored which made the space look enormous, particularly with the twelve-foot ceilings. I placed an Art Deco bar against the mirrored wall. Separating the living room from dining area was a stunning, faux elephant tusk console with glass top. So even though it was no where near finished, it looked impressive to the boy from Addison, Illinois—another obscure suburb.

"Your place looks like a museum," I took that as a compliment.

Seated on the sectional we made small talk. His Mom was a waitress. She worked hard. His Dad drove a bread truck and drank beer. After finishing a 6-pack, he would walk into Jeff's room and show him his right hand and say, "See this? My right hand is my best friend." Without another word, he would leave the room.

Did I need to learn that on what was really our first date?

We talked about music. Bands I had never heard of. And, at some point, he asked if I wanted to see his tattoo. I reminded him I could not see. Hopefully, soon, but not yet. Not now. He forgot and gave me a hug. I hugged him back and all of the sudden a voice in my head repeatedly told me, "Go to first. Go to first!"

And we did.

That's when my tongue discovered he wore earrings. More than one in his right ear. Not that I was against them, but I always imagined me with a LaSalle Street kind of guy—if I were to be with a guy. You know, designer suit and tie from Bigsby and Kruthers or Sir Real. White button-down shirt with collar stays. Lace up dress shoes. No earrings. Not in 1984. Now everyone wears them. Jeff was not the LaSalle Street guy. However, he was awfully nice. I thought so when his friend

Athena first introduced me to him. Should I let his tattoo or earnings cloud my judgement? That seemed hypocritical.

We talked every day. Well, he did most of the talking and I did most of the listening.

The following week I underwent the cataract extraction. It was relatively simple although I stayed in the hospital overnight. With the help of a hard contact lens, I could see much better. I did not have a lens implant. If ever I need additional laser treatments, that would need to be surgically removed which could infect the eye.

Today this is done as outpatient surgery.

Dr. Fetkenhour confirmed the vision in my right eye was miraculously 20/25. I would take that any day. However, there was a new problem with my left eye. Scar tissue formed causing the retina to pull away from the macula which provides the sharp, central vision needed for reading, driving, and seeing fine detail.

I permanently lost the vision in that eye because a large area of the retina tore down the middle. Since I had good vision in the right eye, and the now-blinded left one moved in harmony with it, there was a greater chance of more damage resulting if he were to operate. He recommended doing nothing. No more surgery. Unless *something happened.* Almost forty years later other doctors have told me the same thing. Do nothing. The same risks still exist.

I decided my vision was good enough to drive out to the suburbs. Wearing a big furry, nearly floor-length, double-breasted stadium coat, I met Jeff at a suburban hotel. The coat was Nutria. It cost a fortune but was a business expense.

I was young and needed to look uber successful to convince potential clients that I knew what I was doing. Jeff spotted me immediately and ran to greet me. I reached out to give him a hug—one he didn't accept. He's allergic to fur. We had a fast dinner and then saw *Friday the 13th: The Final Chapter*. We both love scary movies.

The following week I invited Jeff, Sue, her husband Tom, and another couple over for Christmas. We put up a tree in my living room and ordered pizza. Wrapped in holiday cheer, both couples thought Jeff was adorable. The jury was out.

John Dunphy preferred life in the suburbs and rarely came to his home in the city so I bought his share of our building. It upset me. We had known each other for almost 10 years. That was 40 percent of my entire life. I didn't have any other friends who went back that far. Well, except Leana.

Jeff moved in between Christmas and New Year's. He brought his clothes, a lot of CD's and VHS tapes with him. One music video was by a new artist from Michigan. Jeff said she was going to be big. He knows how to pick them. Her name is Madonna. The rest is history.

THE PARTY'S OVER

Things were not going the way we hoped in Texas. Mom suspected my father resorting to his old ways, just a new dress size. One morning she decided to take a detour on the way to her office. Knowing it was Dad's day off she stopped at Chick Smith Ford, the car dealership where he worked.

When the owner spotted her through his office windows, he jumped up to greet her. "Jean, what are you doing here?"

"I came to pick up some papers for Ray." She tried to be convincing as she continued toward his office.

"I didn't know you came back to Spring (Texas) after your daughter's wedding..." Cindy also moved to Texas with her boyfriend. My whole family left me for Texas. But then Cindy and her John (not a pimp—the boyfriend) moved back to Chicago and got married.

Mom stopped. "Chick, what are you talking about? That was over two months ago. I returned to work after the wedding. You know, I am the Houston Hertz Lady."

"Ray said you and your pretty little daughter didn't come back with him." Chick, in his black suit, dark tie and Texas-shaped gold cufflinks stood at Dad's office door blocking mother's entrance.

Mom stared directly into his eyes, "Well, you can see Ray forgot. Here I AM. Please move. I have to be at work soon."

"You don't want to go in there, Jean" my dad's silver-haired boss said quietly.

"Thank you, Chick, but yes I do."

Slowly, he moved out of her way.

Mom proceeded into the small office. Two steps in, she froze. On his desk were framed photos of a woman with some kids. Not Mom and not us kids. She forced herself to the desk and stared at them. Her hands shook as she placed them in her bag. Head held high she marched out the door as everyone watched.

Of course, Dad came up with some cockamamie story about the young lady and her kids. Mom wouldn't listen. It was the beginning of their final ending.

Mom and Regina's lives in Texas had no resemblance to the paradise Dad promised as he duped Mom into marrying him a second time. They only saw Dad when he came home to shower, change clothes, and sometimes eat a meal with them.

In both marriages, Mom managed the money. She could stretch a dollar from Chicago to St. Louis when necessary. So, when April's bills arrived, she scrutinized the monthly stack to determine they were not being overcharged or double billed for anything. That month's American Express statement included a curious invoice from a local furniture store. She immediately phoned the retailer to question the mistake. There was not one piece of new furniture in her house.

After describing the situation to a clerk in the store's accounting department, her call was transferred to Sally, the salesperson who handled the transaction.

"Ma'am, is your husband The Duke?" Sally asked.

"What?" Mom fumbled. "Uh yes. Yes, he is." She forgot the stupid nickname he was given at Chick Smith Ford.

"Why, I remember that sale, Ma'am. Your husband came in with your daughter and granddaughter. They were shopping for furniture for her new townhouse. They spent quite a bit of time here looking at everything before making up their minds..."

"Did they now?"

"Yes'm. And in the end, he didn't spare one nickel, the Duke didn't. When they were done, he said he could get me a deal on a used car so I'm gonna go on over to Chick Smith Ford and check 'm out."

"Well, isn't that nice?" said Mom. "I'm sure he will git you a good deal. Will you be working tomorrow?"

"Yes Ma'am..."

"Sally, ah haven't seen the furniture in my daughter's place yet. Haven't had any time y 'know. It would be easier for me to stop bah you. Ah'm sure it looks better on the showroom floor. Would you be able to show me everything, so I could pick out some accessories?"

"I would love to. And maybe I could help you find some new things for your home too..."

Mom did an Academy Award-winning job of concealing her fury. She was angry with herself for working and trying to stretch the money Dad gave her. Obviously, there was more than she knew. Mom was even more outraged with herself for marrying him. Twice. Once was enough to get the four children she loved and adored. And she hated Texas. It was a long way from their family and friends. She wanted to go home.

On her lunch break, she met Sally at the furniture store. Carefully examining each piece my father purchased for their alleged daughter and her little girl. That lying sack of shit. When they finished looking at everything Mom confided her suspicions to Sally who failed to exhibit surprise. In fact, she told Mom he and the woman (who turned out to be younger than my sister Cindy) were too friendly to be in a father-daughter relationship. She asked what she might do to help. If Mom needed a witness in court, Sally volunteered to take a day off to testify.

Three days later the store delivered half a truck load of new furniture to Mom's house. It was not the prettiest she had ever seen. In fact, it was God awful. She instructed the movers to pile everything in the living room. Literally. When they offered to move the existing furniture into another spot or put it in the garage, she refused asking them to stack it in the middle of the living room.

"Thank you kindly."

When the men left, Mom went to the garage and looked at the tools on the wall. It was the moment she anticipated since her furniture shopping spree, even though the thought of wasting so much money hurt her.

It took both hands to grab the Husqvarna 50 Rancher chainsaw from the wall. As heavy as it was she managed to haul it into the house.

The power cord took several tugs before the engine roared. Having started Grandpa Niemec's pink fishing boat motor many times this was a piece of cake. When she finished, sawdust and bits of fabric flew through the living room. She intentionally left pieces large enough for my father to recognize. Not sure how he would react, Mom locked the orange bodied chainsaw in the trunk of her car and did the same with his guns.

Mom told Regina the story when she returned from school. My sister's face lit up and she began laughing when she ran into the living room. The dust had not finished settling.

"He's gonna be so mad."

Mom nodded. While they could hardly wait for Bad Daddy to show up, Mom scoured the yellow pages in search of a divorce lawyer. She'd had it.

A few hours later his car pulled into the driveway. Regina was at the kitchen table doing homework. Mom was washing dishes. They heard the Duke's cowboy boots hit the hardwood floor when he entered. Had they run a marathon, their hearts could not have beat faster. Waiting. He stopped at the entry to the living room for a long minute, then slowly continued to the kitchen.

"What's for dinner?" he asked, seating himself.

"We already ate. You should go to your girlfriend's home and ask her," Mom replied.

He crossed his arms over his chest and stuck one leg out from his chair. The tip of his cowboy boot pointed towards the ceiling.

"Why do you have a girlfriend?" thirteen-year-old Regina asked. "What's going on? Don't you love us anymore?"

He said nothing. Following a long uncomfortable silence, Dad rose and left the house. Mom sat next to Regina, put her head down on the table and wept.

During the next few weeks, Mom and Regina planned their future. Renting an apartment in Texas was an option. The cost of living was less than up north. But Regina did not want to stay. As soon as school let out they headed home.

WHAT'S UP DOC?

The first year of any relationship is always difficult. Getting to love the good and learning not to hate the bad. One month after Jeff moved in with me, he packed up his things and left. Why?

I wouldn't let his three-foot-long Chinese Water Dragon live with us. If I loved Jeff, I should love his dragon too. And I would NEVER love that—it ate blind mice. So, he left.

Several days later we started talking again. I missed him. When he didn't want to speak to me, I would talk with his mom. Sometimes for an hour. I told her I missed the smell of his coffee. Even though I wouldn't drink it the aroma reminded me of Jeff. I had one cup my entire life. The acid did not agree with my stomach, so I never had a second cup. That's why God made Tab and Diet Coke! I also missed his scary movies and music. I pleaded with her to tell him to come back.

Two weeks later he returned. He agreed my "museum" was no place for a dragon. It would ruin the furniture. For a few more years he kept it at his mom's house and would visit it faithfully. He did not want the reptile to forget him. Ultimately though, he donated it to the Lincoln Park Zoo. They were thrilled to have it and when we went to check on it in the reptile house, the dragon would spot Jeff and smile.

At the same time, my Sue gave me her notice. Her marriage was on the rocks, and she needed a real job. As a parting gift she took the typewriter with her.

***

While Mom and Regina were still in Texas, Dad made the mistake of driving his boss's grandchildren, not even teenagers, to the Houston airport. They were meeting their father, recently divorced from their mother, at a horse farm in Ireland for a vacation that lasted twelve years. Dad had to testify in front of a grand jury making Mom scared to death someone might kidnap Regina in retribution. Chick Smith's grandchildren's photos were printed on milk cartons while the FBI searched for them worldwide.

When Regina and Mom finally returned, it was quite the shit show. They pulled Dad's sailboat behind their car. Named after his girlfriend, it was loaded with boxes and furniture. Inside the car were suitcases, Mom, Regina, and Brandy—my Irish Setter. The three of them moved into the vacant apartment below ours for the summer of 1985 although Brandy visited Jeff and me often. While I was on an appointment Jeff waited for them with Ray and some high school buddies who were going to unload everything into their new home.

Jeff went grocery shopping and prepared food for the weary travelers before their arrival. He is very generous and kindhearted, which motivated them to immediately accept Jeff as part of our family.

Every night we heard Mom cry. For hours. Hidden away in her bedroom immediately beneath ours. Some nights she didn't sleep at all which was rough as she had to work. Hertz transferred her back to Chicago which was fortunate.

They liked her. They really liked her.

There was no money from Dad. Just her car, the boat, and some crappy furniture.

Mom cried all summer.

To cheer her up, I thought a night at the theater would take her mind off her problems. I asked Ray and Gertrude to join us. We saw *La Cage Aux Folles* a musical about George and his Saint-Tropez nightclub featuring drag shows where his lover is the star. Georges' son, Jean-Michel, brings home his fiancé and her ultra-conservative parents to meet the family. The rest is slap stick comedy sung to Jerry Herman lyrics. Everyone laughed through the entire performance. Everyone but Mom. It was clear she was not entertained when she exclaimed "it's a sin".

It was a hard summer for her.

***

After Jeff and I returned from my third winter holiday with Gertrude in Acapulco I became sick. At first I thought it was a bad case of *turista* even though I never had THAT before. We were always careful about what we ate. Never anything from a street vendor or some seedy restaurant. Finally, I visited my internist Dr. Oyer. He himself wheeled me from his office to the hospital. He said perhaps I just needed fluids though he didn't sound convincing.

Northwestern Memorial Hospital is a teaching institution which should explain why a school of interns swam in and out of my room asking the same questions. How long have you felt this way? What did you eat in Acapulco? (That question had a three-page answer). What did you drink there? (Do I tell them everything?) Why did you go there? (Obviously, they'd never been.) How often do you test your sugar? (OMG. How many times do I have to answer that?) Do you smoke? (No.) Have you ever smoked? (No.) Recreational drugs? (Only a pot brownie years ago.) What kind of medications do you take? (Then a blood pressure pill and insulin by injection.) Have you been hospitalized before? (Yes.) Oh really? What for? (Check your hospital records. All my hospitalizations were here). Family history. Is there a history of cancer in your family? (Yes.) Mental illness? (My family is mental as anything.) High blood pressure? (Everyone over 50.) Emphysema? (My maternal grandfather's brother.) Leukemia? (I don't think so.) Are you married? (No.) Do you live alone? (No.)

More tests. More pokes.

"Pee in the urinal please. We need to track your output. The nurse will come and pick it up later."

Lucky her.

Every day, after work Mom came to visit. She was busy during the daytime selling $200 million annually to Hertz Rent-A-Car corporate clients.

On the third day of captivity Dr. Oyer, returned to see me. He didn't look happy but then, if I were going to see someone who had *turista* I wouldn't be too happy either. He just blurted it out…

"John. The fluids are helping. You were really dehydrated. But you need a new kidney…"

"I need a new **WHAT**?"

Asshole.

I wanted to flick the TV back on to see what Lauren was going to do when she learned "Contemporary Woman" featured Paul as it's centerfold. *The Young and the Restless* offered more upbeat information than my doctor.

Oyer grasped the foot of my bed… waiting for my reaction. After all my eye surgeries and other crap I'd already experienced I don't know what he expected of me. I just looked at him and said "Okay."

That black cloud just wouldn't go away.

In my mid-20s and working feverishly to build my brand as a luxury designer, I had no time for another medical detour let alone something as menacing as a kidney transplant.

How does one find a new kidney?

Obviously, I couldn't phone my personal shopper at Neiman's and ask him to set aside a few for me to try on in the Men's department. But how many points would I earn if I bought one on triple points day?

The next morning the team of doctors and a trail of interns showed up at the same time as my breakfast. While Northwestern was doing kidney transplants, Dr. Oyer did not recommend I have the surgery there. The hospital did not have enough experience. Kidney transplants were still experimental. Instead, he endorsed the University of Minnesota Hospital in Minneapolis. It was where kidney transplants were pioneered, the first ever performed there in 1966. Twenty years later they reported a sixty percent success rate.

Was that statistic supposed to be encouraging?

Mom, Ray and I flew to the Twin Cities to confer with the kidney transplant wizards. Jeff stayed behind with his clients who needed their hair cut and colored. He couldn't cancel their appointments.

I've never been so scared. Well, except for the previous years when I couldn't see. I didn't want to go blind, but I really didn't want a kidney transplant either. The chances of dying on this new operating table were far greater than before.

It was all so surreal. I couldn't believe this was happening. Was it a dream? More like a nightmare.

The enormous red brick building's geometric footprint shot out in several seemingly unorganized directions. Its sterile, hard surfaces were cold and off-putting. Far too much fluorescent lighting throughout the corridors and laboratories made even the doctors and nurses look sick.

Mom was more overwhelmed than I. She thought kidney failure something some unlucky 50-or-60-year-olds might experience. Ray took notes diligently. We soon learned even small children, babies, needed and received transplants. We all wondered how they fit a father's adult-sized kidney into an eighteen-month-old baby's body.

My evaluation lasted several days. A group of doctors and nurses had to determine if I met the University's requirements for transplantation. Was I healthy enough to tolerate surgery and the lifelong post-transplant medications? Did I have any medical conditions that might interfere with transplant success? Would I cooperate and follow the suggestions of the transplant team?

Accepting the news about the kidney transplant made me crazy, but then they suggested I consider a pancreas transplant too. They just started to "experiment" with them and would I like to try one?

I didn't know if I wanted a kidney transplant and they wanted to sign me up for a pancreas. I was already freaking out about the possible failure of the procedure. I didn't need to add pancreatic panic to my insanity.

Many different blood tests were performed. They took more blood from me than an Anne Rice vampire. Diagnostic tests including a cardiac stress test, chest X-rays, ultrasound, kidney biopsy were done to evaluate my overall health. Plus, bladder and urethra urodynamic testing. Psychological issues regarding the support I would receive from my family and Jeff—I had to tell them about him—was assessed. They questioned the stress in my life.

Who wouldn't be stressed out while anticipating an organ transplant?

The medical team and social workers who thought they were helping only made me more anxious. The out-of-pocket expenses for a kidney transplant including doctors' visits, blood tests, prescription drugs, hospital room charges, surgery, other related procedures and, in my case, air fare, hotel, rental car or cab fare and food would be around $143,500.00. In 1986 that was $30,000.00 more than the average cost of a new home in America.

I needed a valium. A 10 mg one.

Six weeks later, Dr. Oyer delivered the news—I was accepted for the transplant. Early intervention was not then part of the protocol. My end stage kidney failure had to progress to almost fatal severity before surgery would be scheduled. Oyer said he had no idea how long it would take for my kidneys to fail. When they did, I would probably need dialysis prior to the surgery.

My entire family stepped up to the transplant plate. They were evaluated to determine who had the closest tissue and blood type to qualify as a living donor. The tests also ensured that neither the donor nor recipient carry antigens which might adversely influence the transplant. Cindy was a perfect match. Ray a close second. Mom was third. Being in her mid-teens, Regina was ruled out. Bad Daddy was also tested but not a match. *I knew that.* If I didn't look so much like him, I would have thought I was adopted.

Mom quickly resolved the issue. Provided the doctors agreed, she insisted on being the donor. Reasoning neither Cindy nor Ray had families yet, she argued someday they might be faced with needing to donate a kidney for a child of their own.

"If I am not cheating John of a better kidney from someone else, I want to give him one of mine," she told the doctors.

At the time, the life expectancy for a transplanted kidney was 12 to 15 years. The doctors proclaimed her a perfectly fit donor.

Waiting was the worst.

After being confirmed a transplant prospect there was nothing to do but wait. Wait and wonder. Would this work? How long would it take? Would I survive? What would life be like after transplantation? I rode a physical and emotional seesaw. Besides feeling rotten, every hour of every day was filled with fear and apprehension. Yet, I didn't dare let my clients know how I felt. I worried they'd feel sorry for me and then make up an excuse about not being able to continue with their projects. Rather than dwell on the situation, I worked like a madman.

Against both Mom and Jeff's advice, I sold my three-flat in Chicago's trendy Bucktown neighborhood. It was unfortunate the sale occurred way before the neighborhood became popular, but I still made more than double what I invested in it. Immediately, I purchased another building also needing to be gutted and rehabbed to hopefully force appreciation. In my pre-transplant days, I desperately craved distractions.

On a secluded short street directly behind a hotel, a block and a half from the lake, the location was a step up from my Bucktown digs. The three large apartments had hardwood floors, fireplaces, lots of fine-looking moldings. There were two spacious bedrooms, a formal dining room, sunroom, and large kitchen with butler's pantry. It included a six-car garage which I counted on being demolished by one of the hotel's supply trucks while maneuvering the sharp turn at the alley's corner.

Unfortunately, that never happened.

Continuing to immerse myself in work, I convinced a former uncle, a builder of handsome custom homes, to turn a spec house he was constructing into a designer showhouse to benefit the American Diabetes Association. He agreed and I obsessed over the gorgeous dining room I committed to creating.

Careful to shield my deteriorating condition from my growing list of valuable clients, I sandwiched business meetings, installations, interviews with design editors and more between frequent blood tests, transfusions, constant monitoring—and a bout of toxemia. I threw up every morning. Diseased kidneys lose the ability to remove protein waste so I could no longer eat chicken, beef or pork. My salad and blanched veggie diet grew tiresome, but I didn't have much of an appetite for anything other than surviving.

Each day, after Mom left work, she came home to another job—determining alternate ways to keep me alive.

"What about a pilgrimage to Medugorje?" she asked.

The hamlet in Bosnia-Herzegovina. Healing miracles have allegedly taken place on a spot where six children reported having conversations with the Blessed Virgin Mary. An estimated 30 million pilgrims visited there since the reputed apparitions began in 1981. Some recounted numerous physical healings ranging from cancer to brain disease to multiple sclerosis.

Could I be the next miracle?

Another time our conversation turned from progress of the new building to Mom declaring "We should go to Bucharest."

The drug, Gerovital, was developed there as a "cure all" for a huge range of human ailments. Reportedly taken by John F. Kennedy, Marlene Dietrich, Kirk Douglas and other celebrities—the US banned its importation and sale in 1982.

But should we consider it?

Mom was relentless in finding options to save her first surviving child, but ultimately, we decided not to risk miracles or cure-alls. We opted to go with modern medicine and the sixty percent factor.

In November, a writer for a Chicago newspaper asked how Jeff and I would decorate our new home for the holidays. She wanted to feature it as a Christmas story. I planned on doing nothing, but her call motivated me. Over the long Thanksgiving weekend, we filled our home with much needed Christmas cheer. Lots of it. Thinking this might be my last one we decorated three trees and hung a deer head above the fireplace. When the photographer arrived, my feet were so swollen from toxemia I couldn't wear shoes. Also, my skin was turning a pale shade of yellow. In one picture, I stood behind the dining table so only the upper half of me was visible with two trees dressed in holiday attire.

Shortly after the story ran, the most amazing thing happened. I received a phone call from a prospective client asking if I could meet him and his wife. He wanted to discuss an estate he had recently purchased saying their new home was a gut job.

Music to my ears.

Sick as a pig, I was intrigued and exhilarated. I would have the kidney transplant. All would go well. Then I would return to this commission.

To prepare for the meeting I stayed in bed for two days with my feet propped up on a pile of pillows. I had to reduce the swelling to wear a decent pair of shoes.

They were a lovely couple. The purpose of the meeting was for them to determine if they liked me. It was a short meeting. I wasn't sure I "sold" myself since they graciously dismissed me. On my way home I beat myself up wondering what I did wrong. I wanted this job so badly.

The next day, after I finished throwing up, I went to my desk and moved papers from one side to the other—not able to concentrate on anything.

The phone rang. I wasn't in the mood to talk to anyone, but I picked it up. "John Robert Wiltgen Design."

"Yes. Is John there?"

"Speaking."

"This is John Blaney. I am sorry about last night. Mary Louise was not feeling well but we want you to work with us. When can you start?"

See. It's true. The Lord giveth and the Lord taketh away.

He was giving me the Blaneys and taking away my kidney. That's life. I had to learn to roll with the punches.

I said I was leaving soon for my annual winter holiday in Acapulco and asked if we could start when I returned. That was fine with them as they were also going away.

***

January 2 my mother and I flew to Minneapolis. Two warriors riding into battle. Needing a kidney structure exam, I needed to be hospitalized a couple days prior to surgery. Like any responsible transplant patient, I prepared for my check-in by visiting the nearest tanning salon. When we returned to Chicago, I had to appear tan and rested—ready to tackle this newest commission.

My hospital roommate was an irritable old man who just received his kidney transplant. He swore I would wish I were dead by the time the surgeon finished. He wished he were dead.

I wished he were dead.

I worked so hard at preparing myself mentally for transplantation. But at that moment my roommate totally fucked up my emotional coolness and the most powerful fear overwhelmed me. I wondered, once again, why me? What did I do to deserve kidney failure?

I mean, besides eat everything I shouldn't?

Did I want to have a transplant? No. I wanted to go home and die. Really, I wanted to die. I thought I was ready. That's how afraid the old fart made me.

***

January 6, 1987. I don't remember much. On separate gurneys, Mom and I were transported to the operating room together—holding hands. The drugs we needed to sleep for the next eight to ten hours were already administered through our IV's. The last thing I recall is Mom saying she loved me. I replied saying, "I love y…" and was out.

The surgeons and nurses could have done anything to me… to us.

Getting a transplant without having dialysis treatment first is called a preemptive transplant. That is what I had. At the last minute it was determined I did not need dialysis. I was so happy. For whatever reason, I was more afraid of dialysis than the transplant. I did not want my blood pumped through tubes in and out of a machine. The thought of it freaked me out.

Many thoughts freaked me out.

The surgeons placed Mom's kidney in a different location than my original kidneys' which were not removed. They are only removed if they're causing severe problems (kidney failure is not one of them) or are enlarged significantly. The artery delivering blood to the kidney and the vein carrying blood away were surgically connected to those already existing in my pelvis. The ureter was connected to the bladder. Mom's kidney is in my lower abdomen.

The miracles of modern medicine. I was already the benefactor of this and other miracles and I did not have to go to Medugorje.

RECYCLE KIDNEYS
NOT JUST
DIET COKE CANS

My eyelids fluttered briefly. The lights were blinding. Doctors and nurses in pale green scrubs hovered over me. The guy at the foot of the bed didn't have a long black cloak or scythe so I knew Death hadn't come for me.

Thank you, God.

I went into that deep drug induced sleep again. The next thing I knew, the nurses began getting me up to a cacophony of beeping noises. Out of bed. On my feet. A familiar voice. Foggy but familiar. Jeff. He was there. In my room. Helping the nurses. They did not want to risk my developing pneumonia. Jeff said Mom's transplanted kidney worked right from the start. I was peeing up a storm.

The crazy shit we talk about when in the hospital.

With a catheter that emptied into a disgusting plastic bag, an IV for food and drugs, oxygen mask and bandages for days they carefully laid me back in the bed. Again, I escaped far away by means of the deep sleep.

Cindy and Jeff came to Minneapolis the day before surgery. They shared a hotel room which the Hertz Corporation paid for. Mom's sister Aunt Kristine, drove from Tomahawk, Wisconsin with Bradley, my 4-year-old cousin. They brought Grandma Niemec. Ray had just started his job in St. Louis and couldn't be with us. Neither could Regina. She was performing during half-time at the Aloha Bowl in Hawaii with her high school dance team, the Maine South Hawkettes.

Dad came too. On one occasion Cindy was grateful for his presence. She nearly escaped becoming a patient herself the first time she saw Mom after surgery. The sight of our mother tethered to tubes and machines overwhelmed her. Mom's roommate, a dying nun (not a flying one), made the uncomfortable scene worse. Walking into the room, Cindy felt lightheaded. Suddenly, everything turned black. A strange acrid odor (Mom later called it "the smell of death") strangled her. She staggered from the room and fainted at the doorway, falling right into Dad's arms. He saved her from hitting the cold, hard flooring.

She was always Daddy's little girl.

Two doctors who saw Cindy collapse, quickly sat her in a chair and took her vitals. They rushed her to the hospital's outpatient clinic for a thorough exam. After the once over by more doctors, they concluded Cindy was in perfect health. Just stunned and still shaky.

After that, Mom's doctors wasted no time moving her to another room. Even though Mom has always been a profoundly religious woman, they feared her health might be compromised by coping with the stress of a constant stream of grieving sisters praying and clicking their rosary beads as the nun's life ebbed away.

The next day I was walking. I didn't leave my room, but slowly, carefully, anxiously, I made it around my bed as Jeff held me up and the nurses tried to keep all the hoses untangled.

Question after question tumbled through my mind as the pain medication wore off.

What happens now? Will the kidney continue working? Will I reject it? Will the anti-rejection medicines work? How will they make me feel?

Mom's first post-surgery memory was awakening as Jeff wiped her face with a warm towel. He stayed busy running between my room and hers.

"John was up and walking already," he told her.

When Jeff and I strolled into her room together she cried tears of joy despite the tubes protruding from the generic backless hospital gown.

While elated by the apparent success of the transplant, her recovery was much more difficult than mine. She entered the hospital in perfect health. Now she was in tremendous pain. The operation was much tougher on her. Like a magic trick the surgeons cut her in half. They went through the muscle in the lumbar region and removed the tip of a rib to retrieve the kidney for me. From her belly button to her spine. Experiencing five C-sections during her child-bearing years left a belly teeming with scar tissue making her healing much more difficult than another donor.

Today, kidneys are removed laparoscopically which has many benefits. It reduces postoperative hospital stays by several days and recovery time by weeks. Back then, the procedure was much more complicated.

Taking the morphine the doctors prescribed for her pain after surgery did not suit her.

"Enough!" she insisted, waving away a nurse who had come to administer more.

Mom asked the nurse to remove a lovely picture opposite her bed. She saw spiders crawling out of its colorful flowers convincing her she needed to work through her recovery without chemical crutches.

With a clear head I was euphoric. Peeing up a storm made me so happy. But my exhilaration began to waver when the reality of my required daily cocktail of anti-rejection drugs set in. Immunosuppressant drugs would help prevent my body from rejecting the transplanted organ, but there was a downside. The university schooled me in the unnerving set of hazards each script presented, before I would be discharged.

Cyclosporine. Back then it came in a bottle with an eye dropper and tasted like motor oil. We were to mix it with apple juice or something sweet to make it somewhat tolerable. "Somewhat" being the key word. It was awful. It made my skin and hair greasy. Other side effects include headaches, diarrhea, heartburn, increased hair growth on the face, arms and back, acne, uncontrollable shaking, burning in the extremities, breast enlargement in men, and depression. It could also cause kidney failure!

Why would they prescribe a drug that caused kidney failure? Today, there is a modified version of cyclosporine in pill form that is less toxic than the motor oil version, although the liquid is still prescribed for certain patients.

Imuran. Patients who take this are at increased risk for lymphoma, skin cancer, as well as bacterial, viral, and fungal lung infections having serious consequences including death which is especially serious if you ask me.

Prednisone. This steroid also suppresses the immune system. Short term it will elevate blood glucose. It can also cause patients to retain fluid and lead to bone loss.

Since my transplant was from a living donor and Mom was a great match, I worked my way down to a low dose of these drugs in a relatively short amount of time. I continue to take a handful each morning and at night but not nearly as many as the first-year post-surgery.

Once released from the hospital I returned each day to be examined and give samples of blood. They were meticulous. Rejection is common, particularly within the first six months and is always on your mind. The chance of losing a transplanted organ decreases over the years, but it can occur at any time. For that reason, every transplant recipient must be able to understand their lab results, check for signs of abnormality and stay in constant touch with their team of doctors.

Leaving Minneapolis, I was excited but overwhelmed. Stricken with a new doubt made me wonder—could I create this new life to be worthy of the miraculous gift I received? I have spent every one of my days on earth trying to make that so.

I CAN ONLY
BE ME

The university transplant department announced Mom's kidney settled effortlessly into its new home. They were more excited than me. Three months later I returned to Minnesota to be inspected. Then six. And, finally on my one-year anniversary. After that, I assembled a team of local doctors to run to in case of an emergency.

At home, the bathroom countertop was covered with an assortment of new drugs. But to be able to eat protein again, though in limited amounts because animal proteins are the hardest to digest, was heaven. And to be able to wear shoes.

Tired of being the secret patient I was ready to resume the role of architectural, landscape and interior designer. The first thing I did was call my newest clients to schedule another meeting. I was back from "Acapulco" and ready to get started. With the remnants of my Minneapolis tan, which was fading quickly, I took my brand-new kidney to start the biggest, most important contract of my then blossoming design career.

I was lucky to be alive and they were going to get the best from John Robert Wiltgen Design. Theirs was a dream project. It was a commission I wouldn't allow my medical condition to jeopardize.

This prominent businessman and his wife purchased an 11-acre estate with a vintage 1910, 13-room, classically detailed Georgian home as its centerpiece.

They knew what they wanted. Update the kitchen, five bathrooms and two powder rooms. Elegantly furnish the 10,000-square foot main house. The grounds cried out for a tennis court and spectacular landscaping in the English garden style with lush green lawns, hedges, and borders of breathtaking flowers, grasses and herbs. And they had no intention of moving in until the last picture was hung. Close to perfection is what they desired. The Great Gatsby is what they got. Several years later they called me back to add another 3,500 square feet to their home.

Within less than one year of living in my newest building and 7 months after the transplant, my realtors found a buyer willing to pay an unbelievable sum for my three apartments and dilapidated garage. I accepted the offer and continued to ponder the idea of becoming a real estate developer.

Sometimes my little real estate deals financed my design business when things were slow. To date, I have moved nine times and purchased many condominiums in developments I worked on with clients. Those I either rented or flipped to make a few bucks.

Jeff and I moved into a two-bedroom condo in the luxurious Gold Coast neighborhood. Our building featured two apartments per floor—kind of like Frank Barbaria's building—only our address was a product of the '60's and not nearly as grand. But the neighborhood was. I loved living a short block from the legendary Pump Room. The Playboy Mansion was across the street. I rented an office in River North, close to the Mart, where JRWD remained for 10 years before moving to bigger quarters. Working as a stylist in a salon on Oak Street, Jeff became a star in his own right. He was an awesome colorist and gave great cuts with texturing sheers and clippers. He liked that he could walk to work and not pay for expensive parking.

Within six months of moving into our new digs, Jeff moved out. He was 30 something and never lived on his own. Ever. No matter how much I would miss him, I had to let him go. It was for his own personal growth.

He rented an apartment four or five miles away, bought a fish tank, a parrot, and some basic furnishings. Oh yeah, and a hairless cat, Kito, which cost $3,000.00. At the time inbred Sphynx cats were extremely rare. He saw the breed on the cover of Connoisseur Magazine and had to have one. This one was even more unique because in time it grew hair.

These cats are known for their extroverted behavior. Sphynx are intelligent, energetic, curious, and affectionate towards their owners. They are like dogs, frequently greeting their owners or whoever is at the door. I went to visit the cat, the bird, the fish, and Jeff often.

***

Skimming a local newspaper, I spied a blurb in a gossip column announcing an upcoming fundraiser for the Better Boys

Foundation. A trip to Los Angeles with tickets to the Academy Awards was among the items in their Ninth Annual Celebrity Auction. I wanted that trip and those tickets.

Jeff wasn't interested in going. His excuse was having nothing to wear even though we were the same size and I owned multiple tuxedos.

I was the successful bidder for the LA/Academy Awards trip and another to Washington D.C. including tickets to the Presidential Inaugural Ball. The wife of the founder of the Foundation introduced herself to thank me. She and I became friendly and *voila*—I was named chairperson of their 10th Annual Celebrity Auction. That catapulted me into a new direction. Feeling blessed to have a second chance at life, it became vital to me to give back.

Meanwhile, eighteen-year-old Regina moved into the second bedroom of my Gold Coast residence. My home became her college dorm while she attended DePaul University. She adored living two blocks from Division Street. With girlfriends, who also had fake ID's, they frequented bars where guys bought them drinks. When she needed wheels, she drove my BMW, which I purchased after my Mercedes was stolen from the 6-car garage I previously owned. Between classes she worked in my office. It was an affordable way to attend college.

I recruited her as my co-chair for the gala. We rounded up a bunch of friends and some of my vendors for our committee. We drafted a producer of the Oprah Winfrey Show who organized the lighting, stage and sound contractors. Using the studio's name, she was also able to obtain some great auction items including a leather jacket from Cher's *Heart of Stone* tour which she personally autographed.

Regina was responsible for selecting the meal we would serve our guests. She met with the hotel director of catering who set up a table for her in the mammoth kitchen. A salad, soup, two different entrees, a few deserts and five wines (two white and three red) were presented. How many eighteen-year-olds are saddled with that responsibility? Perhaps that's how she became such a wine aficionado.

Charity can become addicting.

My friend Elizabeth, who is old enough to be my mother, is sophisticated and socially savvy. I knew she could easily navigate the Presidential Inaugural Ball so we flew to Washington D.C. on January 19, 1989. I had never been to the nation's capital. Didn't take the 8th grade school trip because Mother was too worried about something happening to me even though I promised to keep candy in my pocket. God forbid I should pass out at the Lincoln Memorial or during the White House tour.

As part of the auction package, we viewed the inaugural parade from the windows of a prestigious Pennsylvania Avenue law firm along with Jimmy Dean, former Illinois Governor William Stratton, his wife and a bunch of other politicians I didn't recognize. The location was highly preferable to standing in the frosty crowded street fighting for a glimpse of the new President and First Lady surrounded by a bevy of secret service agents.

The Inaugural Ball that we and 5,000 other guests attended was held at Union Station. As we slipped through the building's replica of the Roman Arch of Constantine, I scanned the massive interior. In awe of the 96-foot-high ceilings and assortment of architectural styles I couldn't help but wonder—from a bedroom in the moldy basement of my family home to a Presidential Inaugural Ball…

How did I get so lucky?

The newly elected President George Bush and First Lady Barbara Bush made their third stop of the evening through a nondescript doorway far away from where Liz and I stood. They took to a large stage and after several heart felt thank yous the President made his first proclamation.

"You can say you saw it first here, a lousy dancer trying to dance with the First Lady of the United States of America."

Then, the President embraced his wife and moved around the stage to the Broadway musical classic *I Could Have Danced All Night*. I am not sure who was leading but when the song was over the Bushes were onto the next ball.

Two months later, Liz and I flew to LA to attend the 61st Annual Academy Awards. As we pulled up to the Moorish Revival-style Shrine Auditorium we watched the red-carpet procession on the TV in our car. Lucille Ball was in the limo ahead of us. She was swarmed by the press as she exited. They followed suit with our car but quickly stepped back after discovering we were a couple of nobodies.

Being in the audience at the Oscars is far different than watching it on TV. On one side of the stage Melanie Griffith and Don Johnson presented Geena Davis with Best Supporting Actress while the other side was being prep'd for the next presentation. I was fascinated by the mechanics of it all and paid more attention to that than those receiving awards. Many guests left their seats at commercial breaks attempting to secure their next role, get funding for a movie, or sell a screen-play. As the show went live again, everyone scurried back to their places.

There was no host for the awards that year. Not that they couldn't afford one. The top one-hundred films for 1988 grossed $3,573,577,161. Walter Matthau introduced Hollywood legends Bob Hope and Lucille Ball. It was her last public appearance. Less than a month later she died of an abdominal aortic rupture.

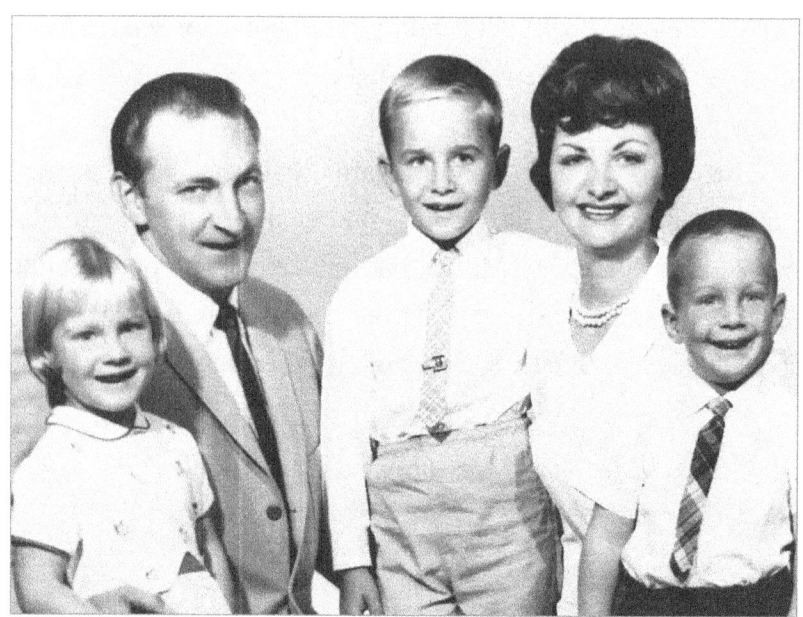

Cindy, Dad, me, Mom, and Baby Ray. We never thought our happy family would be affected by type 1 diabetes.

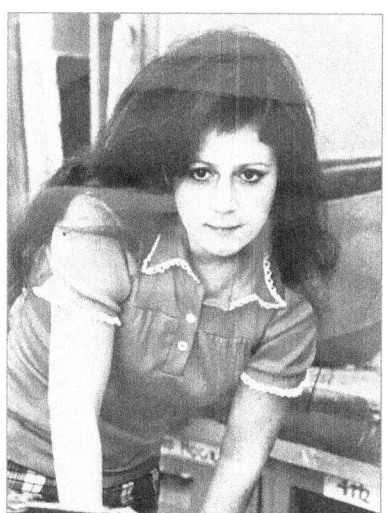

My freshman year art teacher, Ilene Tandalaya Zuckerman. She was my first professional art teacher and provided great encouragement with my art skills.

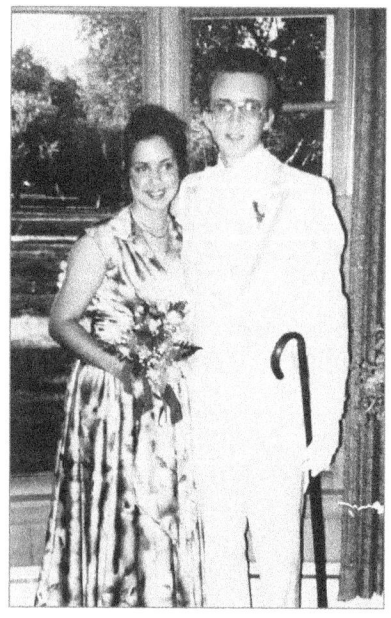

Leana and I on our way to prom. I look so dorky!

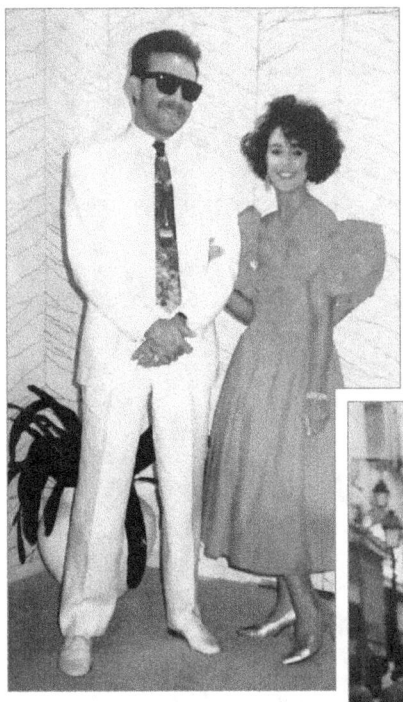

More photos of Leana and I...
Hair from the 80's and this was
my Don Johnson look.

Me with a lot less hair.
Leana and I in Paris.

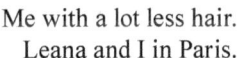

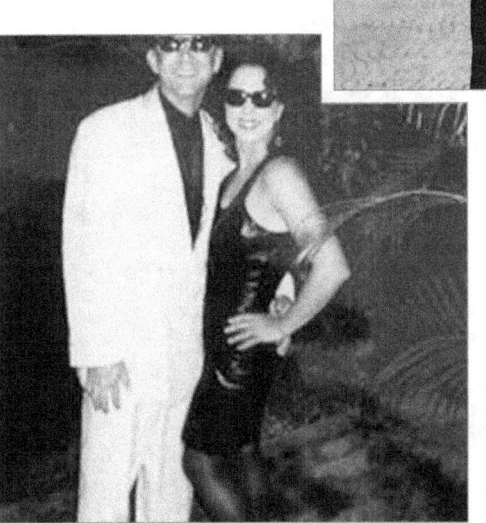

We went to Capos, Costa
Rica. She told me it was
the Riviera of the Pacific
Coast so I ran out and
bought a chartreuse
colored Versace tuxedo.
We were way overdressed!

Jeff and I with my friend Gertrude's housekeeper. Well, condo actually. Minerva worked for Gertrude in Acapulco for more than 20 years and she was like family.

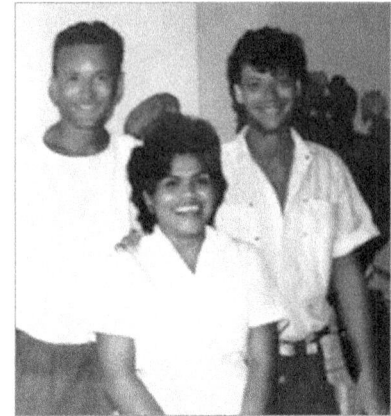

Gertrude and I in Acapulco (below). In the 70's and 80's it was such a great place to escape to.

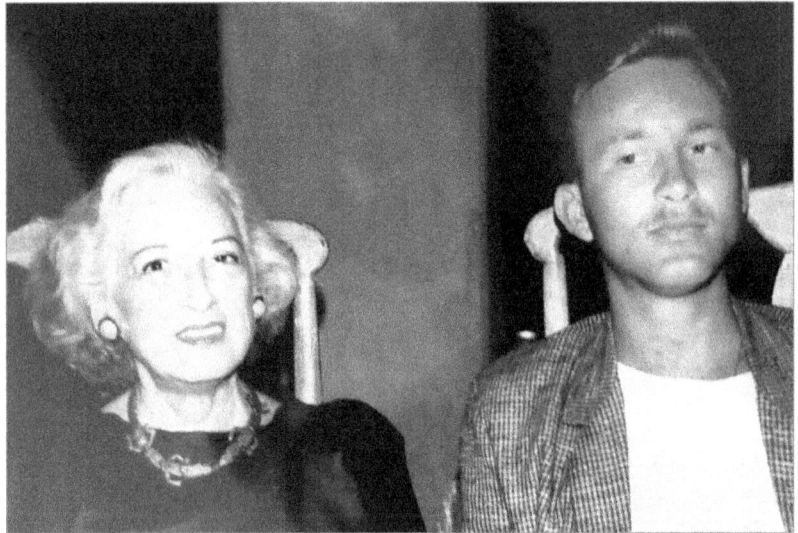

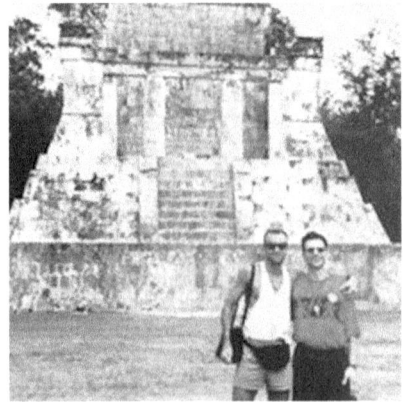

Jeff and I in Coba where the Mayan ruins are a huge complex of temples, pyramids and ball courts. *Why am I so fascinated with all types of antiquity?*

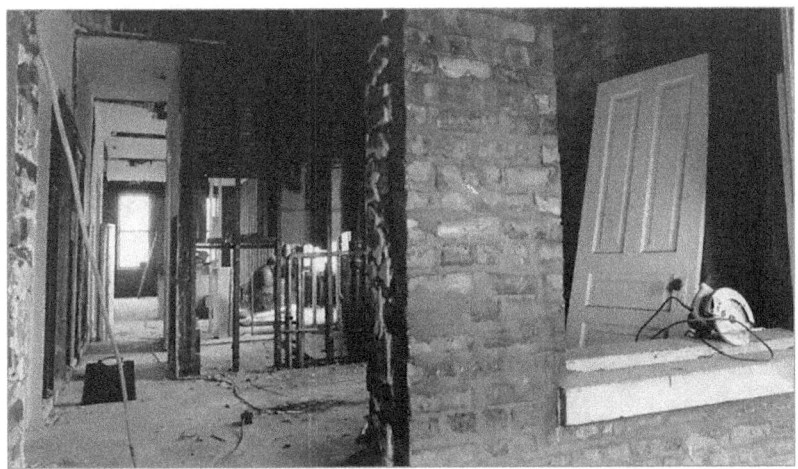

The first 3-flat I purchased when I was 22. Obviously it needed a little work. It took us almost 18 months to renovate. We did a lot of the work ourselves during the time I was fighting retinopathy and could not see.

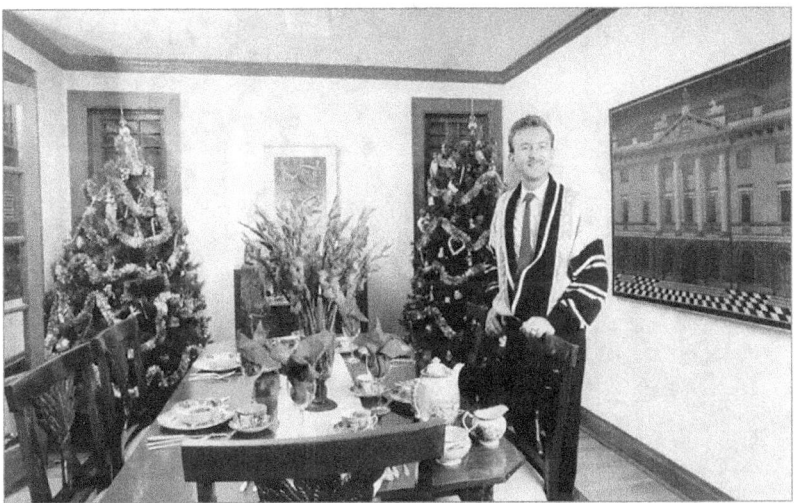

During the holiday season of 1986 I was waiting for my kidney transplant. Not certain I would live to see another Christmas I think I overdid the holiday decorations. There was yet another, larger tree in the living room and a deerhead over the fireplace mantel. When the nespaper photographer took this photo, the swelling of my feet was so bad (from toxemia) I could not wear shoes. Thus, I stood behind the chair. My skin tone was also jaundiced. Good thing the photo was taken in black and white.

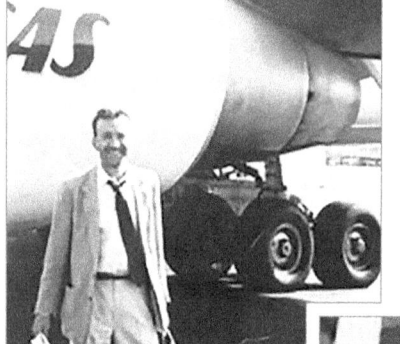

In the spring of 1988, AJ had plans to meet King Olaf in Oslo and asked if I wanted to join her. It was my first trip across the pond and 16 months after my kidney transplant. When we were through, we visited Copenhagen and Brussels.

AJ and I standing in front of the Royal Palace in Oslo. This was not the day we went inside. That evening I wore a Versace tuxedo and she wore a skirt suit with a big slit in the back.

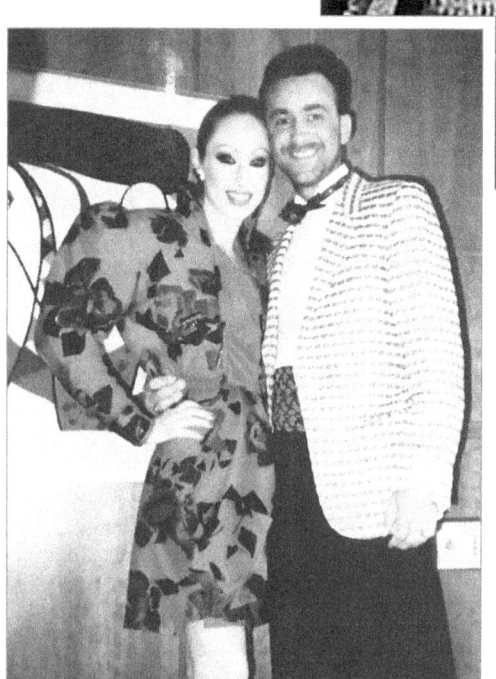

Lara and I in Copenhagen. She was my Faces dance partner before she moved around the world and finally ended up in Kuwait. There she met her Swiss husband Kurt. They have been married for over 40 years

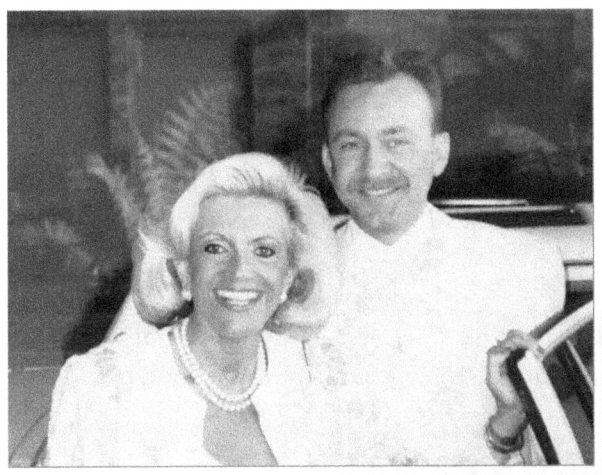

Elizabeth and
I on our way
to the 1989
Academy
Awards.

It was a long and crazy
night.

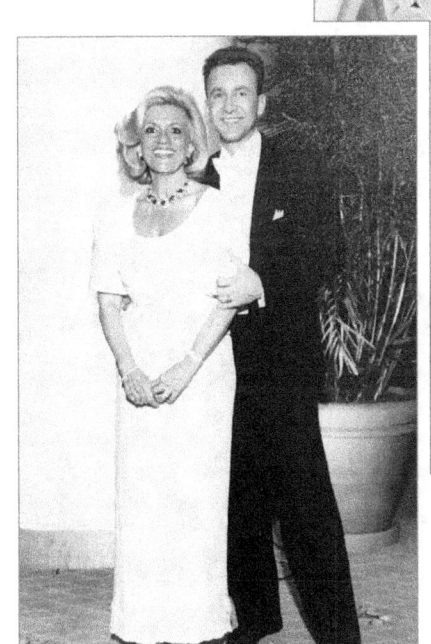

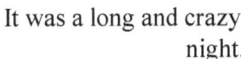

Here we are at the Inaugural Ball.
I shaved off my mustache. Boy
did I look young at this event.

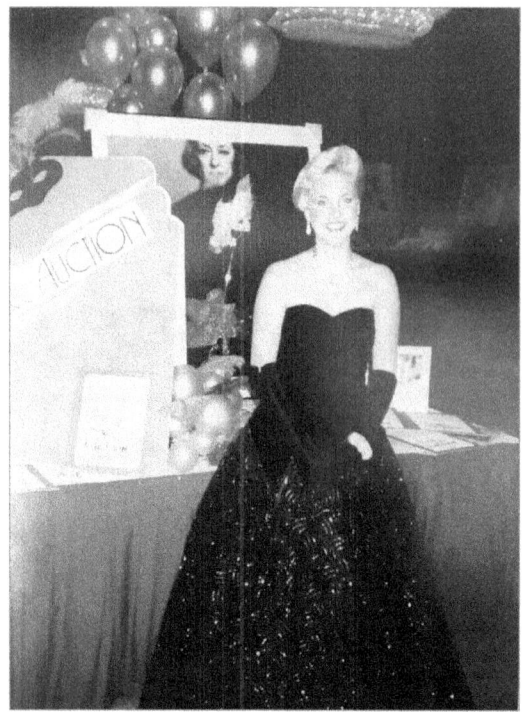

In 1989, my youngest sister Regina and I were the co-chairs of the Better Boys Foundation annual celebrity ball. At 19, she was queen for the night.

The following year we were co-chairs once again. When the lights were dimmed and the indoor fireworks were finished, the spotlights shown on the two of us at the podium. We greeted the 500 guests with "Hi. We're back!"

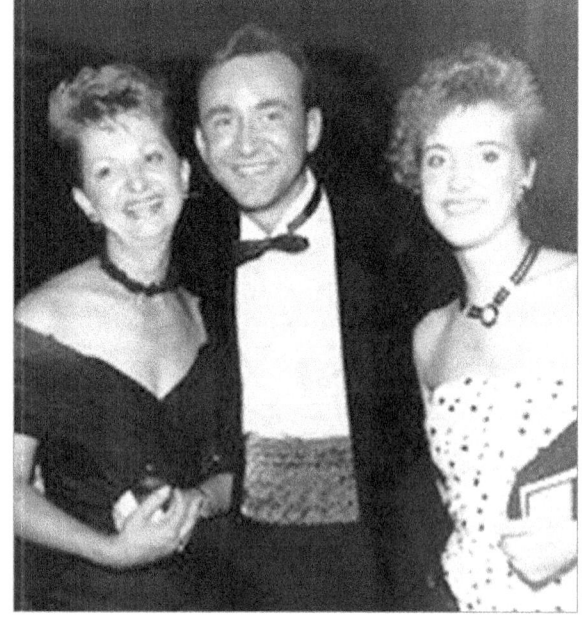

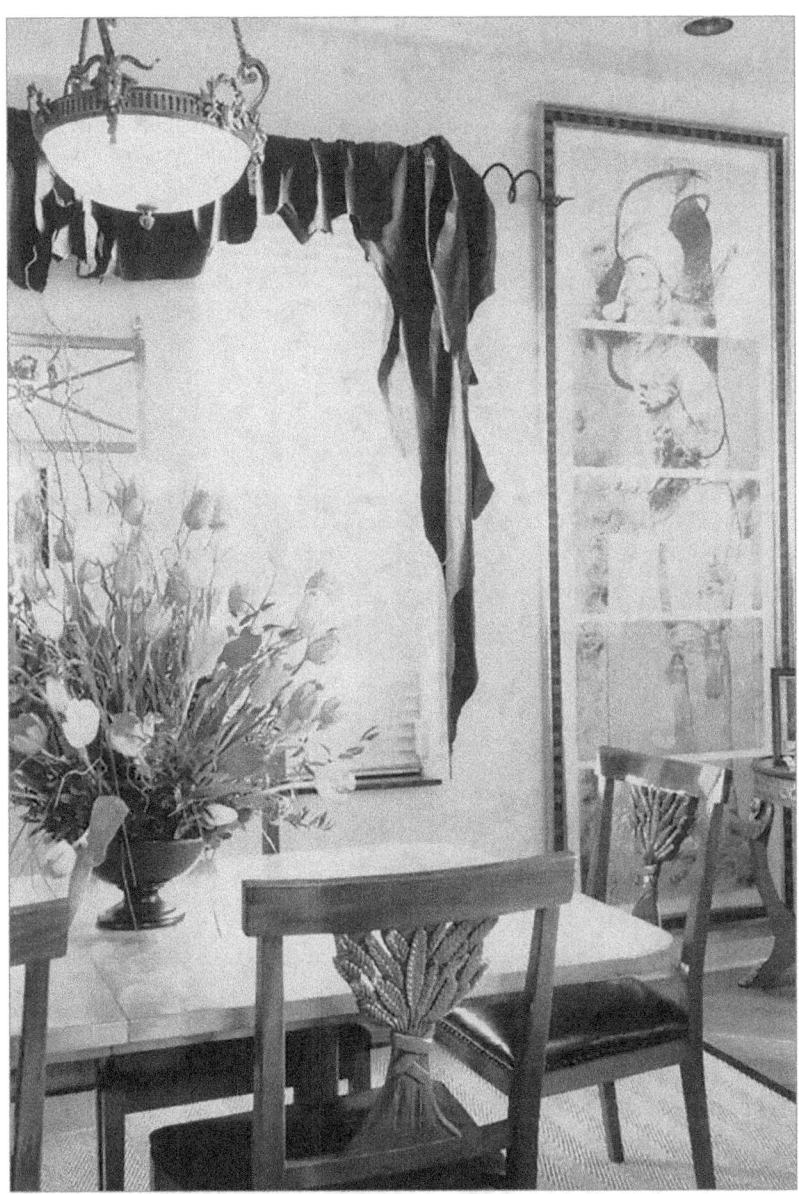

This was my home in the second building I owned in Bucktown which turned into a very chic Chicago neighborhood. The building had 6 apartments. I combined two on each floor to make 3 large, two-bedroom apartments. The living room and dining area had drapes made from leather hides. No sewing needed. I just threw them over a decorative iron rod and voila. My sister-in-law, Gail, thought they were Halloween decorations.

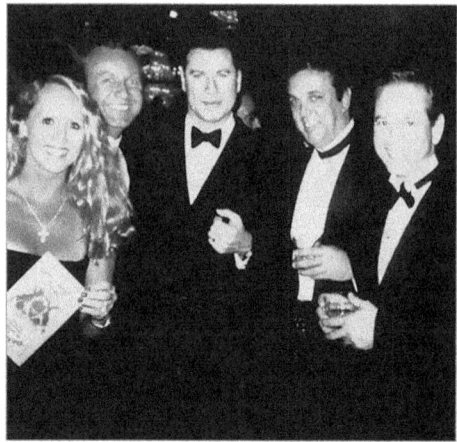

In October, 1998, 1,000 guests were present to pay homage to John Travolta, who received a lifetime achievement award from the 34th Chicago International Film Festival. (From left to right) Karen Murphy a.k.a. Miss Hollywood, me, John Travolta, Bobby Cooper, and Robert Berman. Bobby was in the movie *She's So Lovely* with Sean Penn and John Travolta.

Academy Award-winning actor Tim Hutton received an award for his directorial debut of the film *Digging to China*. We were there to congratulate him. From left to right Timothy Hutton, Bobby Cooper, moi, Georgia Davos and my bf Jeff Meyer.

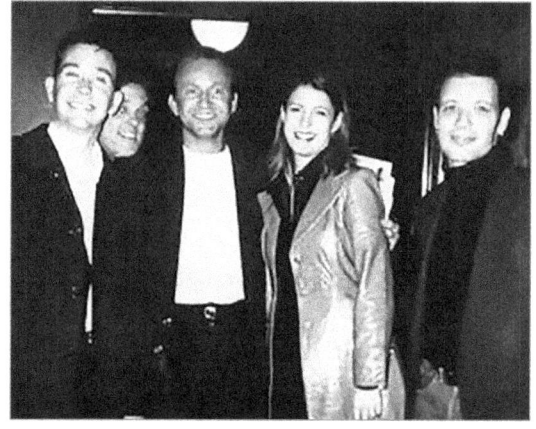

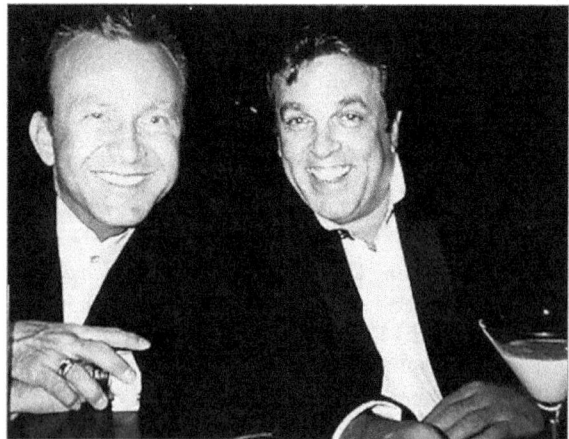

Bobby Cooper hijacked a friend's cell phone. Dialing Sean Penn he ran up to the podium to give John Travolta the phone so Sean could offer his congratulations.

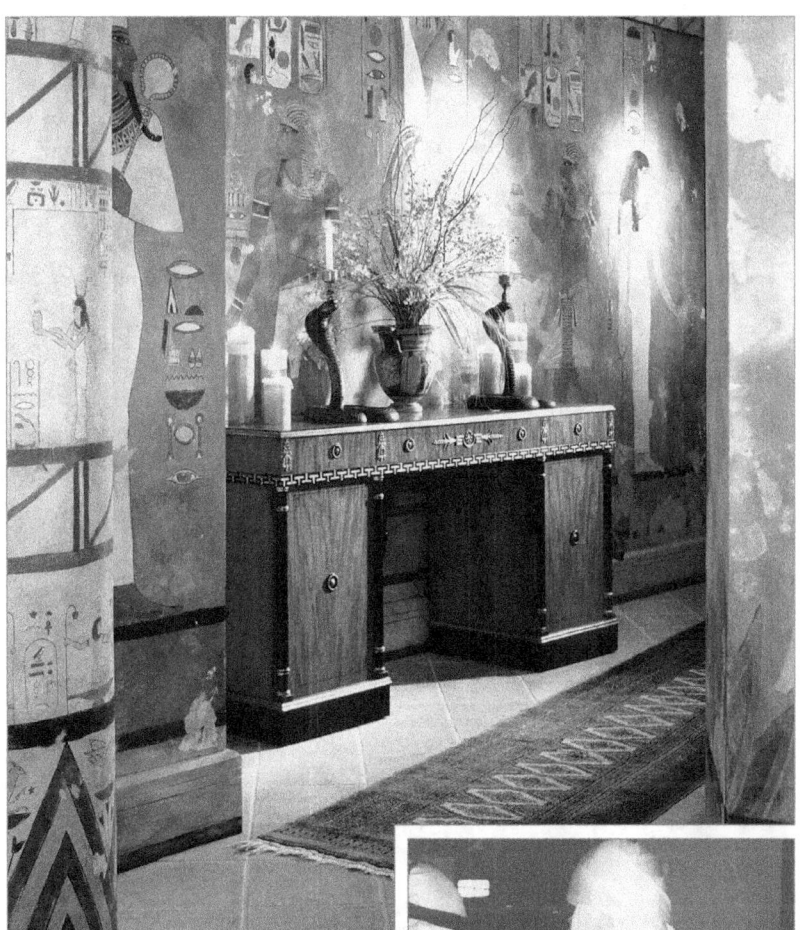

I always had a thing for Egypt.
When I was a little boy, I drew
maps of secret tunnels in pyramids.
When I moved into a loft, I had
every wall painted in hieroglyphs.
The work was done in plaster and
then distressed. That is me on the
right wrapped in gauze. I had to
look good in my home.

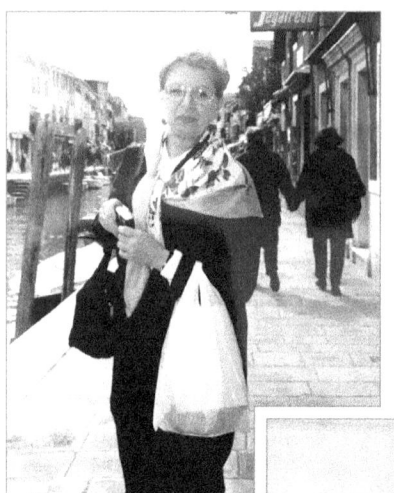

Mom was surprised when the pilot announced we were landing in Venice-on an island! To get to our hotel we took a water taxi. Mom (left) is enjoying our exploration of the city. She looks good for 62, don't you agree? The technology they had 1,000 years ago to construct the 120 individual islands is amazing.

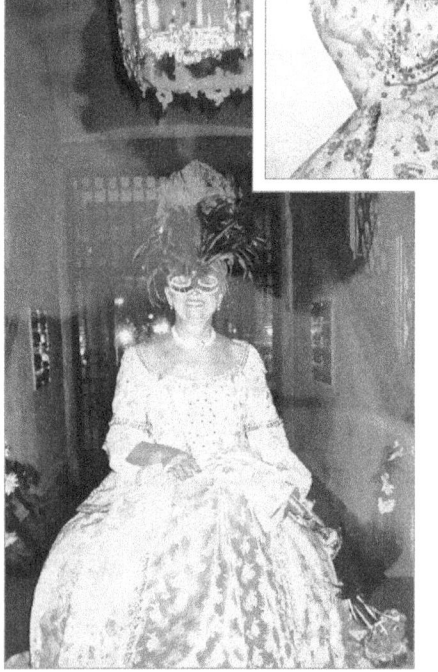

We returned to Venice for Carnavale along with a group of friends. I managed an invitaton to Il Ballo del Doge held in a magnificent palazzo on the Canale Grande.

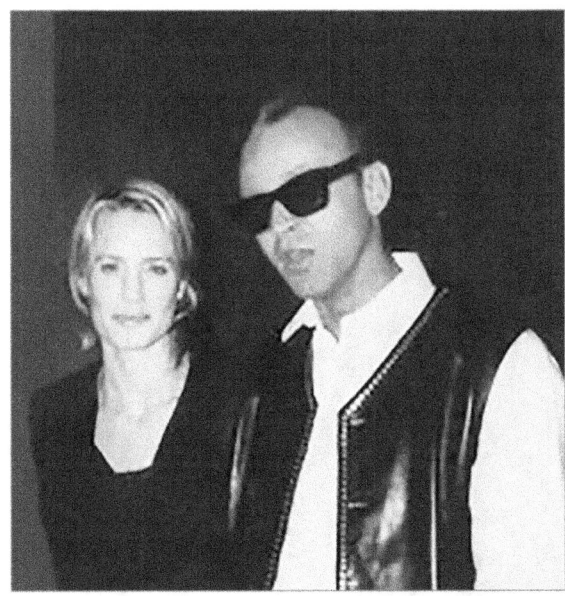

In 1999 *Message in a Bottle* was released starring Robin Wright Penn and Kevin Kostner. Jeff and I were lucky to be admitted into the preview "after" party in Beverly Hills. When it ended we were invited back to Sean and Robin's suite at the Four Seasons.

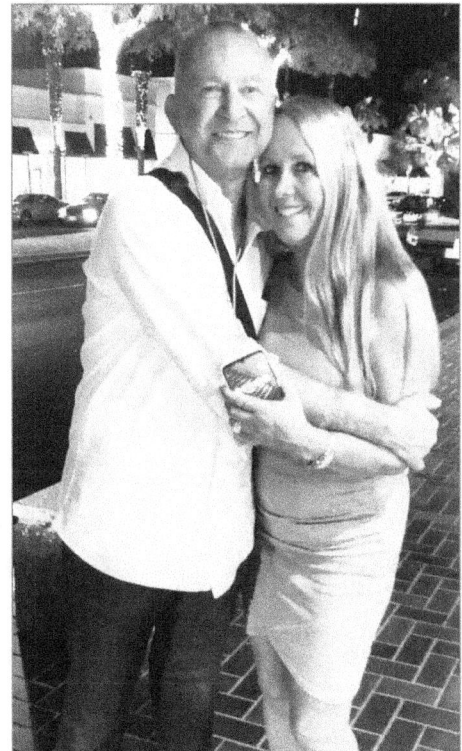

Karen Murphy a.k.a. Miss Hollywood and I on El Paseo in the desert. She is the one who introduced me to some of the A listers of the 90's, their wives and more.

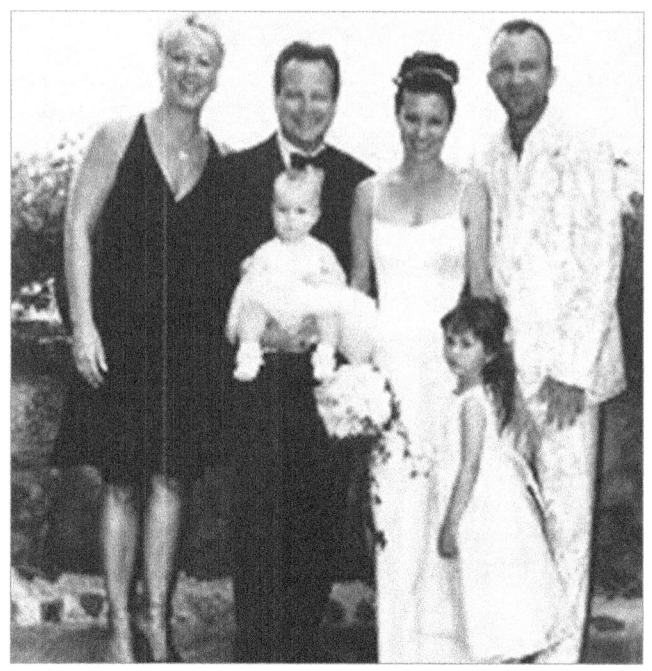

Bill and Leslie's wedding was held in Arrezzo, Italy where the movie Life is Beautiful was made. From left to right: Susan Tjarksen (the Matron of Honor), Bill Senne with daughter Audrey, Leslie Senne with Susan's daughter, Ellie and me.

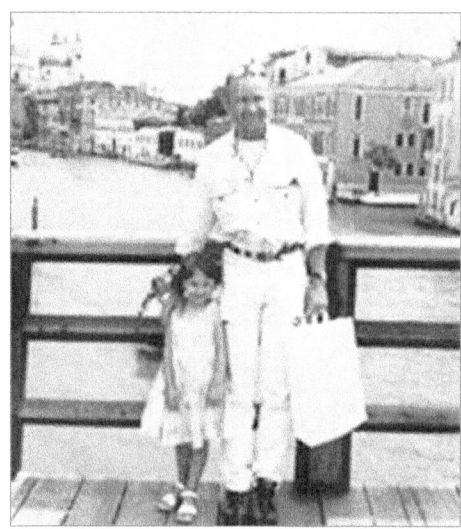

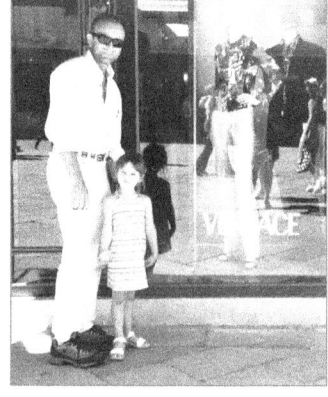

Ellie and me after a little shopping in Venice.

Above: My client and friend Thelma Krause, wife of NBA Hall of Famer, Jerry Krause.

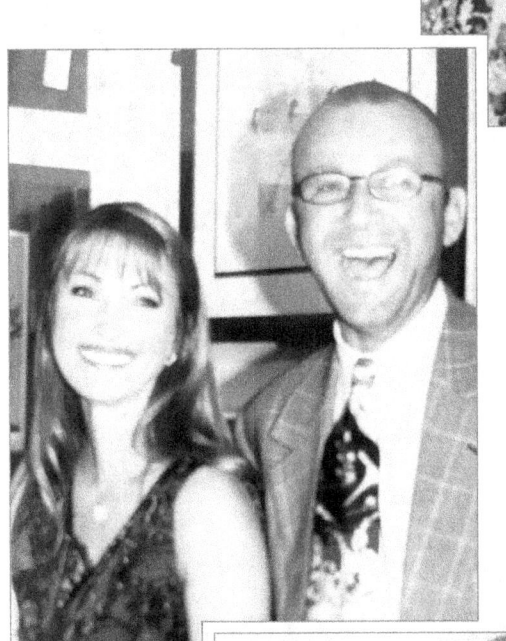

In 2001, after meeting Jane Seymour in Hackensack, New Jersey I hosted a party featuring her artwork. This was put together on a short schedule. Nonetheless, over 300 people attended. Made me think of my middle school days when I wondered what kind of job I would need to be able to host parties.

Not only is she this lovely to look at but she is this lovely on the inside.

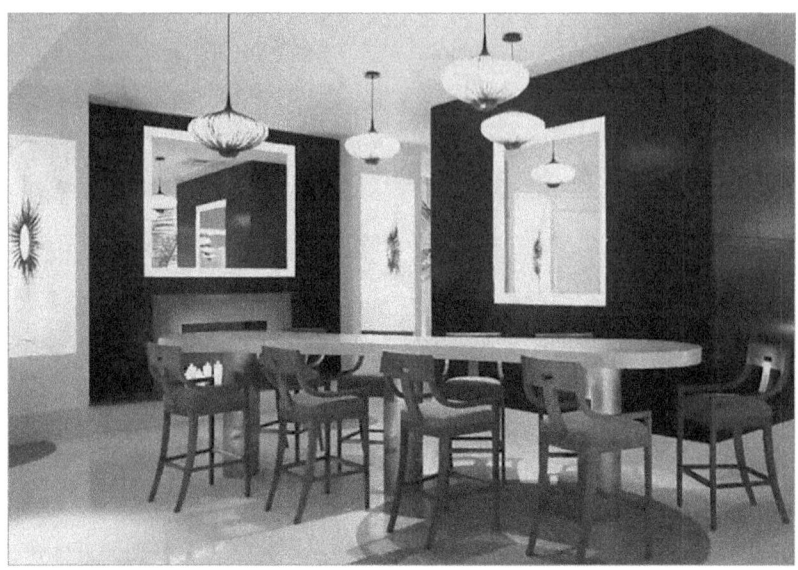

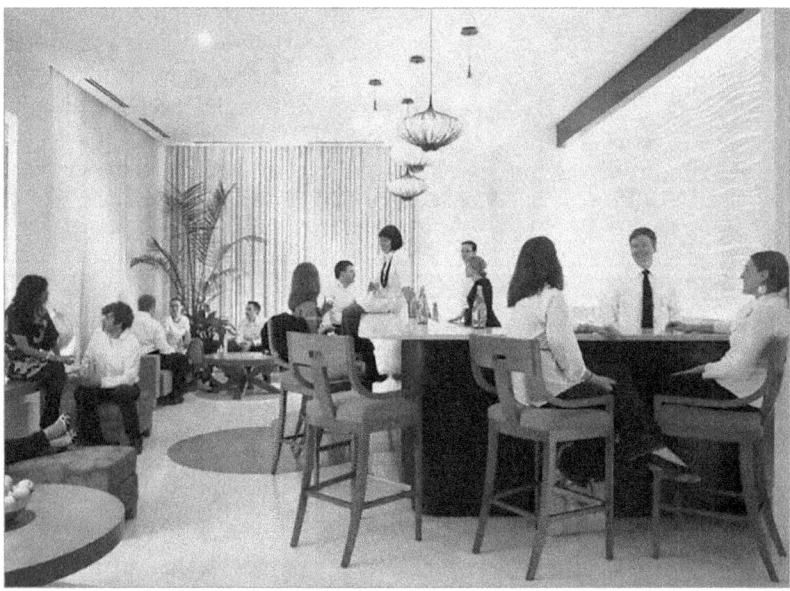

In 1996 John Robert Wiltgen Design, Inc. created an 8,000-square-foot lobby that won numerous awards. Not only was it stunning but it was environmentally friendly. It featured glass terrazzo floors, furnishings made from sustainable woods, recycled polyesters, and decorative silk light fixtures using LED lamps. We were given the raw space and contracted most of the build out with a few exceptions.

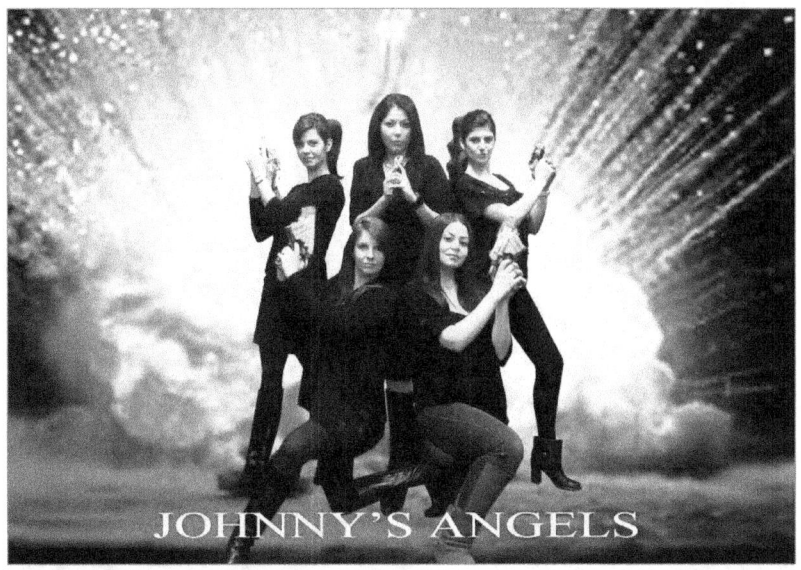

JOHNNY'S ANGELS

The ladies in my office created this photo montage for me. From left to right my angels include Ruxandra, Julie, Maxine, Lisa and Daniela.

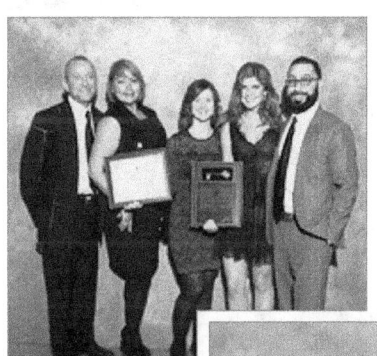

It was rare for me to show up at an awards banquet. When I attended it seemed we didn't win. 2015 though was a good year. From left to right are me, Maxine, Amy, Daniela, and Frankie.

At another awards event- one I did not attend-are Julie, Daniela, Maxine and Ruxanda.

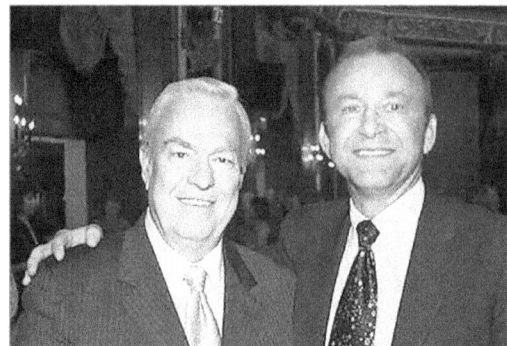

In 2009, the Chicago Academy for the Arts named me the recipient of the Irv and Essee Kupcinet Leadership Award. Television journalist Bill Curtis and I.

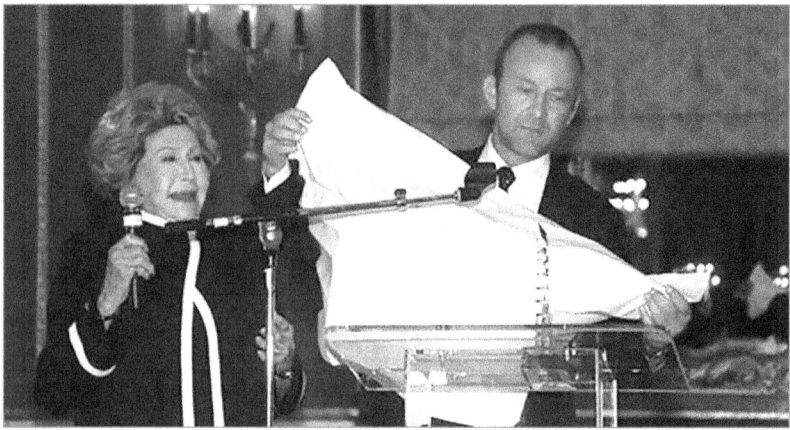

Since my aunt, Bea Levi, flew in from Palm Springs to present me with the award, I had to share it with her. After all she introduced me to the school and pleaded with me to help raise money for it.

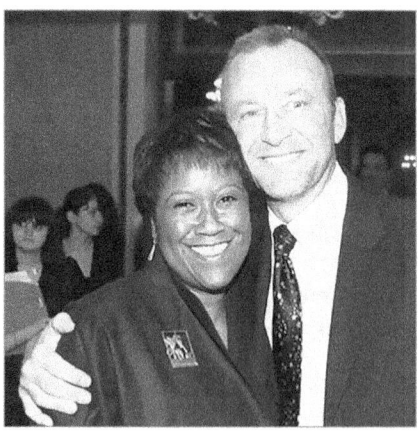

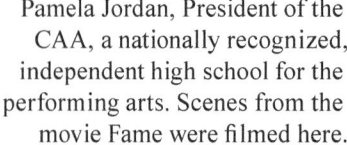

Pamela Jordan, President of the CAA, a nationally recognized, independent high school for the performing arts. Scenes from the movie Fame were filmed here.

Cynthia Rowley, Susan Ester Waccholz Bertendshaw Hauge and I have been friends since I was 17. Susan is the person who saved me and John Robert Wiltgen Design when I could not see.

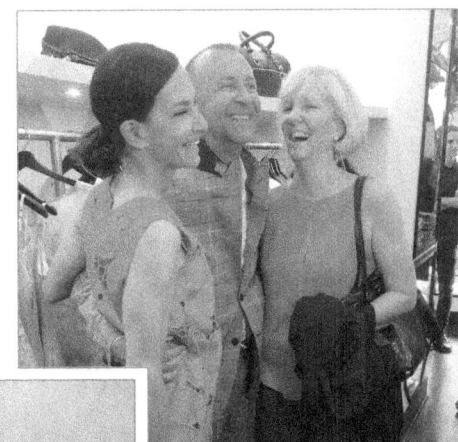

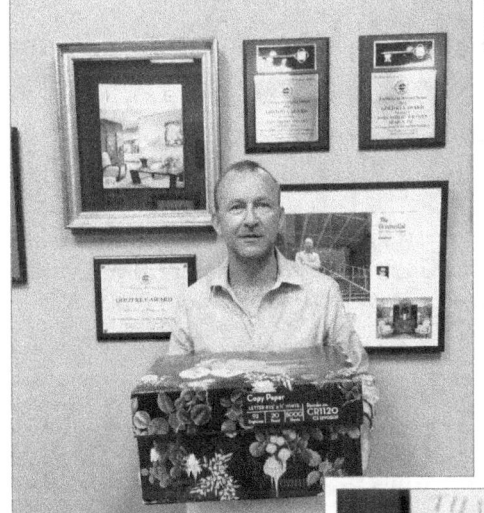

Me in the conference room of my office with a box of Cynthia Rowley printing paper. I had a stapler from her office collection too!

The three of us attending an awards ceremony for Cynthia at the School of the Art Institute of Chicago. Both ladies are alumni of the private art school.

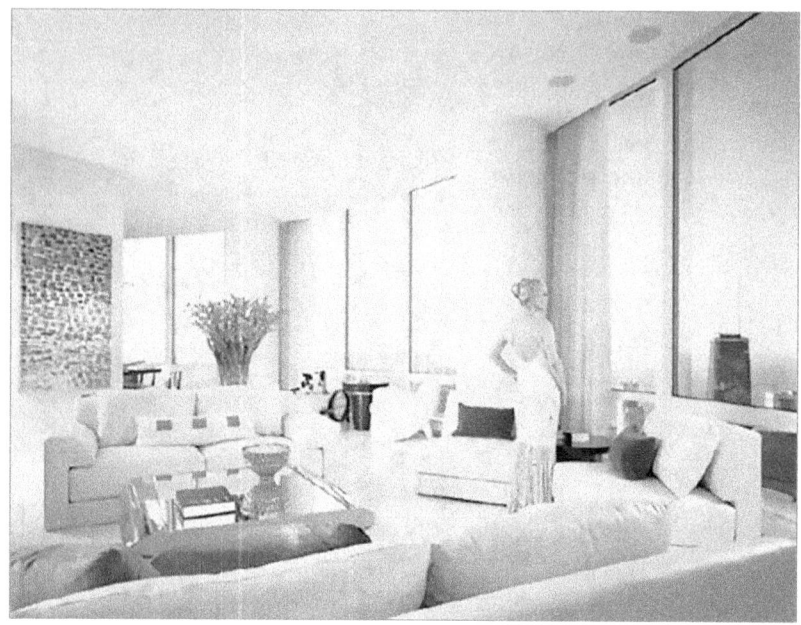

This is the Chicago penthouse project that ultimately took me, my brother, and Susan Tjarksen to Lagos. The US State Department warned Americans of travel to Nigeria but my client lent us two of his armed body guards. Were we nuts or what?

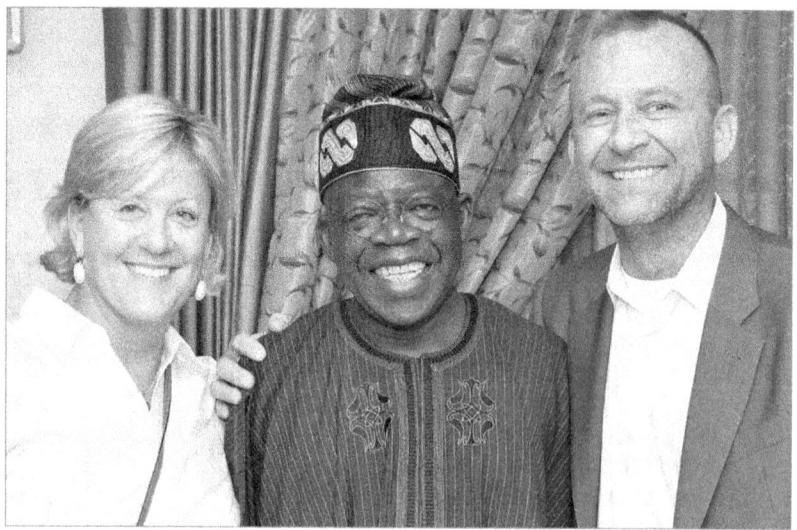

Susan and I with my client, Bola Ahmed Tinubu, the Asiwaju of Lagos (a title given to him by the King meaning "the Leader").

Ray and Fola in the pool. The freestanding poolhouse is 6,000 square feet.

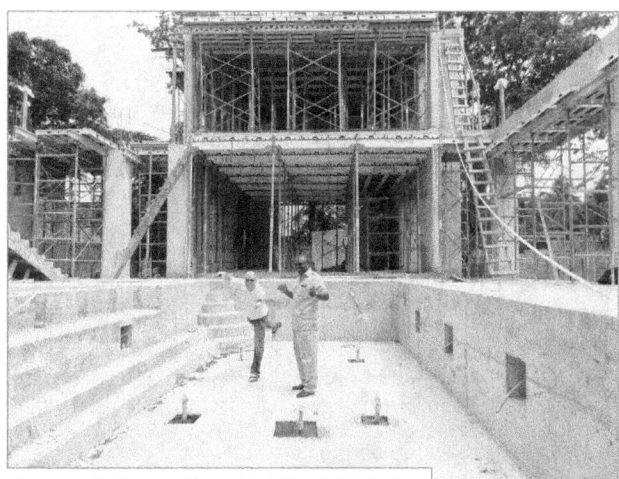

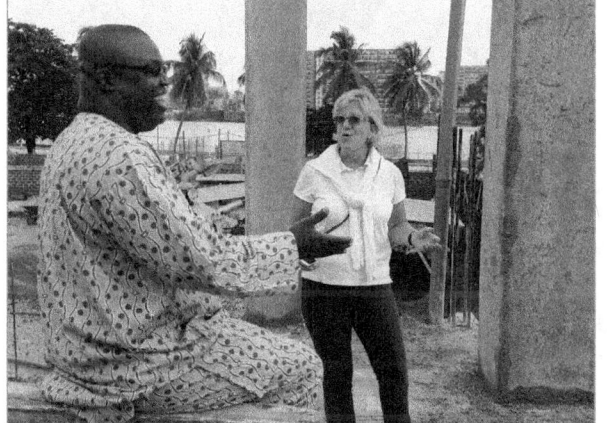

Susan and Fola on site. The harbor, which empties into the Atlantic, is across the street.

One of our visits to Iga Idungaran, the official residence of the king since 1630 to see His Royal Highness the Oba, Rilwan Babatunde Osuolale Aremu Akiolu. During these trips I usually had a PIC line so I could take IV antibiotics to fight cellulitis osteomylitis.

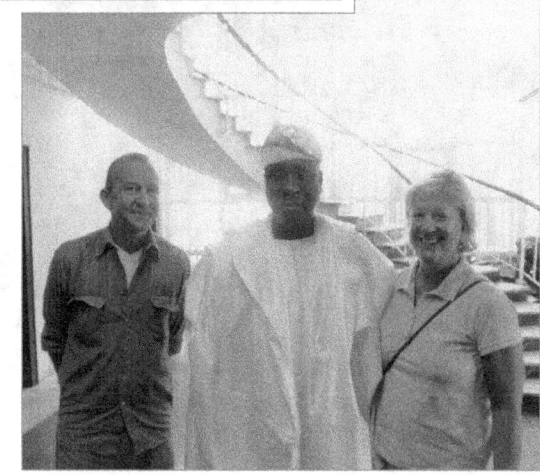

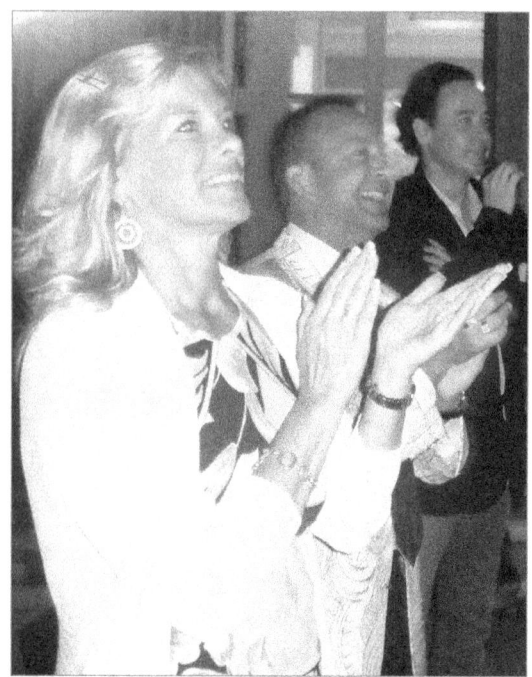

I hosted a farewell dinner in the lobby of the palace at the Kempinski Palace Hotel for my friends and clients who traveled all the way to Istanbul for my "pool" party. Before dessert we watched the fireworks over this magical city. Pictured here are Cheryl Hoban, me and John Cusack.

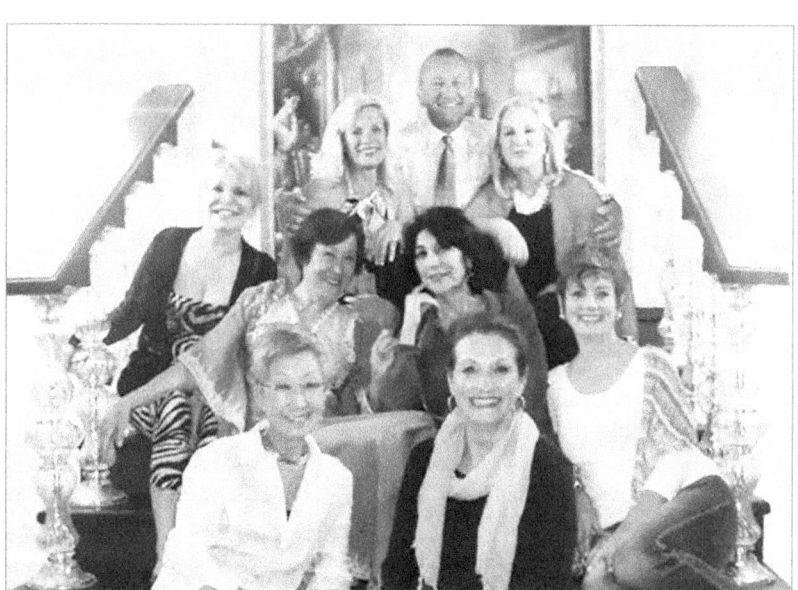

My harem. From top to bottom, left to right. Me. Cheryl Hoban, Tere Proctor, Alice Loftis, Yuriko Byers, Marie Carlson, Dora McDonald, Kiyoko Binosi, and Anna Balice.

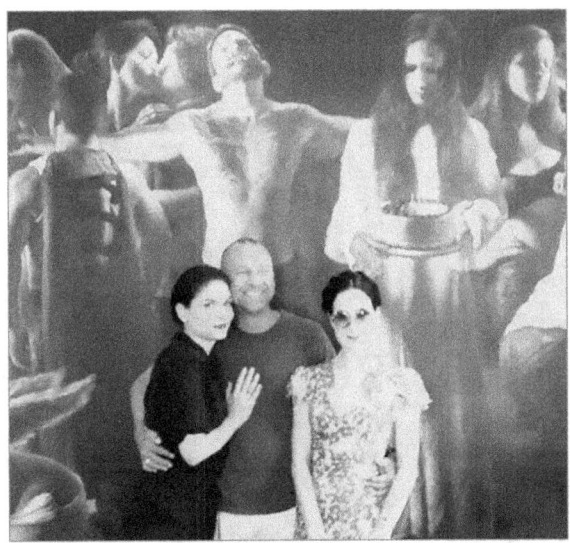

By 2012/2013 the renovation of our new home was complete. Another condo at Metropolitan Place, but this one was larger and had a terrace. Above, actress Jodi O'Keefe and Dita Von Teese visited on a Sunday afternoon.

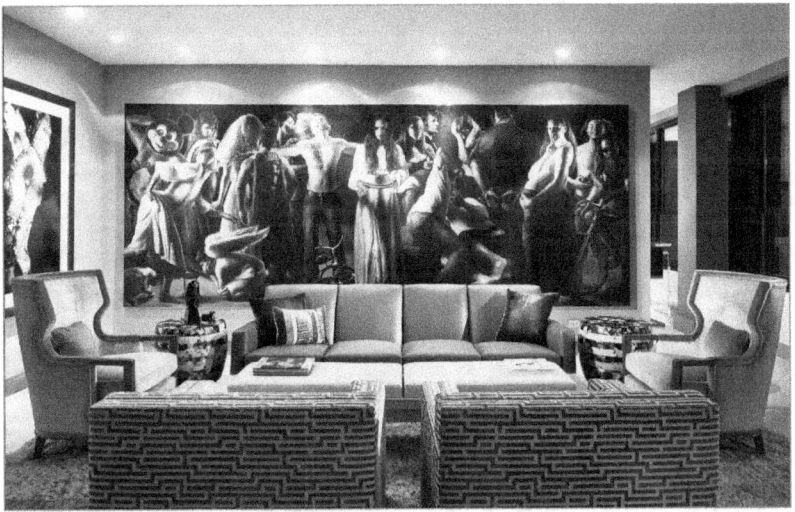

The living room featured an enormous painting by Bruno Surdo entitled Life. It was 17'6" long x 6' tall. Each time someone came over and studied the painting, they saw something new in it. The artist's ability to render all the different textures and his composition were amazing.

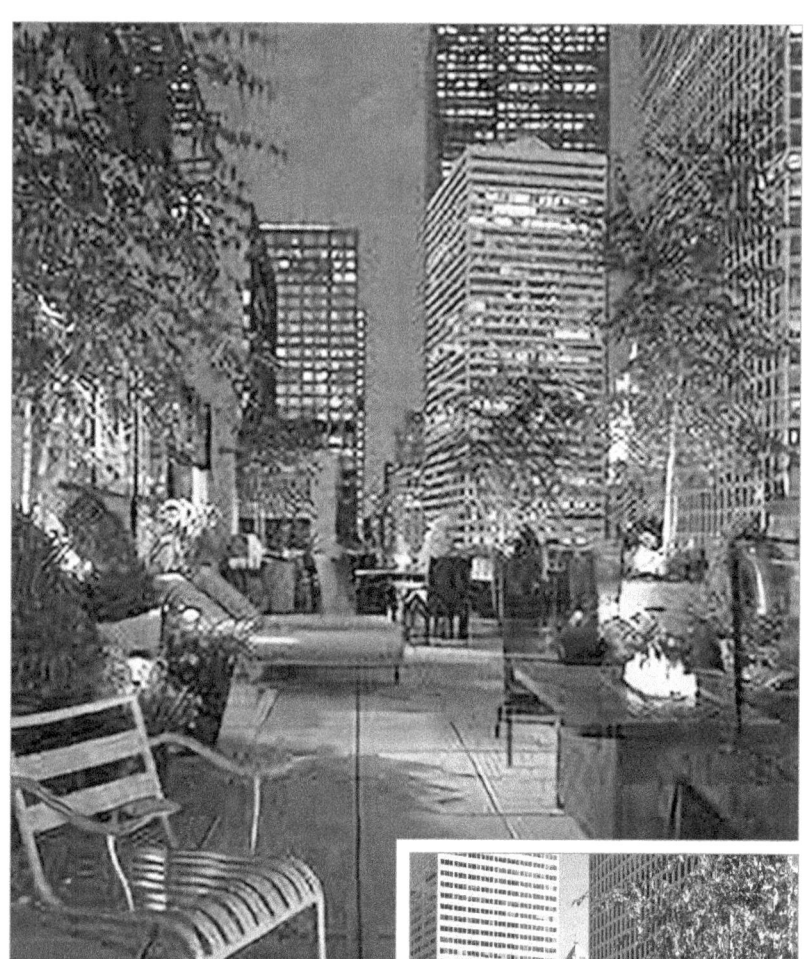

An enveloping southern exposure offered the tranquility that nurtured both our guests and the verdant landscape on our terrace. Through our sliding glass doors it was an inviting escape. The city's hard edges were softened by the lush plantings.

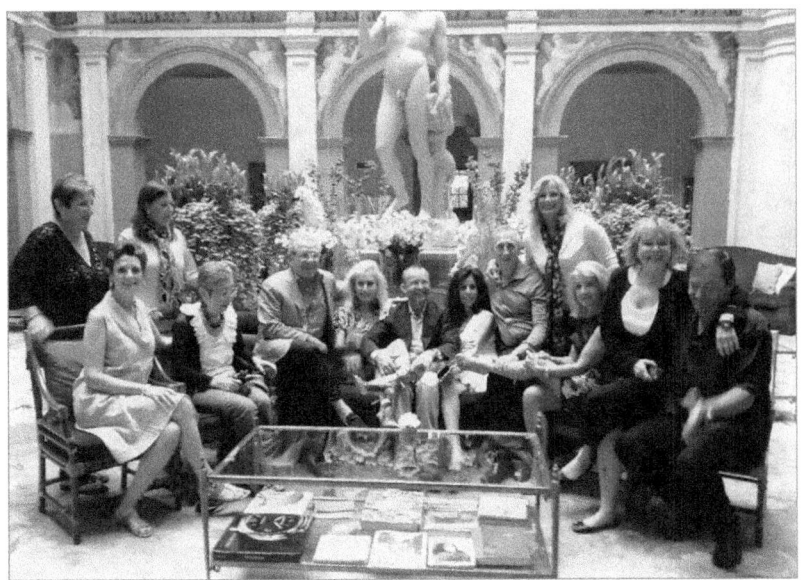

In 2013, 6 months after receiving my first prosthetic, Steven and I hosted a "pool" party in Florence, at the Four Seasons, which was originally a Medici palace.

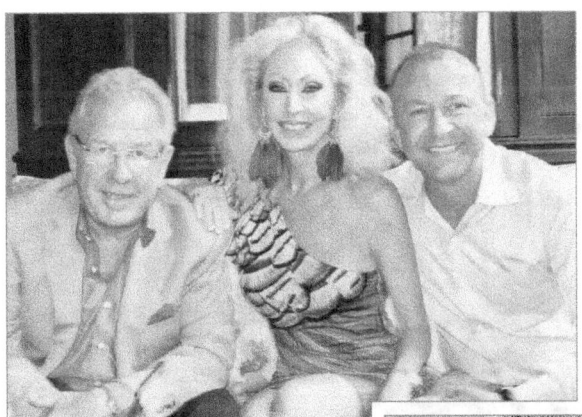

Kurt and Lara came from Switzerland. I was so happy they joined in the fun.

Having a large pool on the hotel grounds is a huge bonus if you are planning a "pool" party. Not many hotels in Florence do. The pool is warm and set amidst the beautiful 11 acre garden.

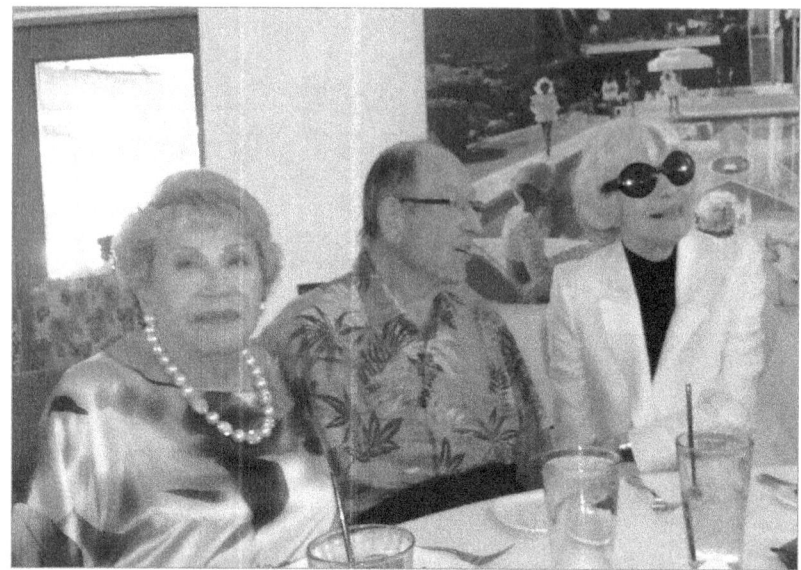

Bea's 90th birthday party was a full week's celebration. Lunches. Dinners. Bea is on the left, her boyfriend Dr. Joe King is in the middle, and Carol Channing is on the right.

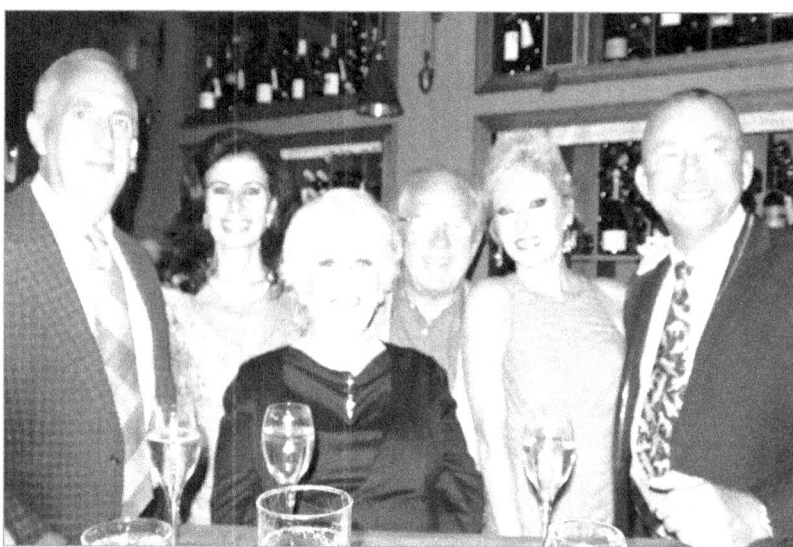

In 2014, our "pool party" started in Zurich and ended in Lake Como. Steven and I were surprised when our friends met us for dinner. From left to right Steven, Diana Sherrer, Rhinda Ensley (Lara's mother), Kurt Ritter, Lara Ritter, and moi. This was the best part of our trip.

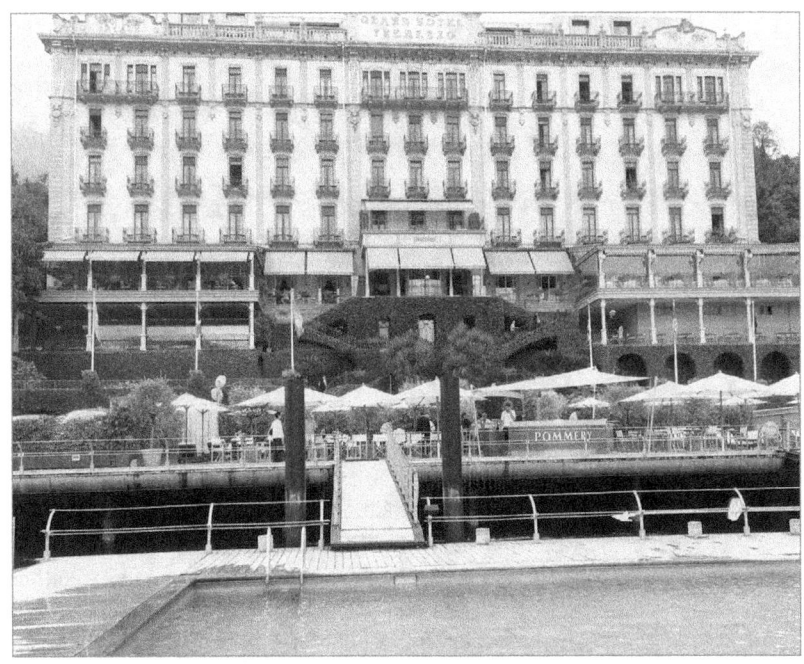

Everyone stayed at the Grand Tremezzo Hotel. The pool floated in the lake on pontoons.

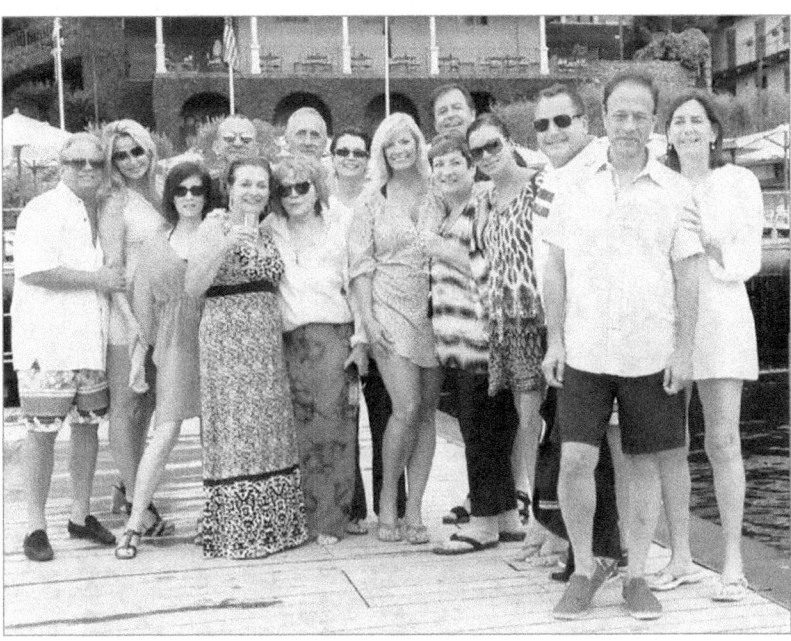

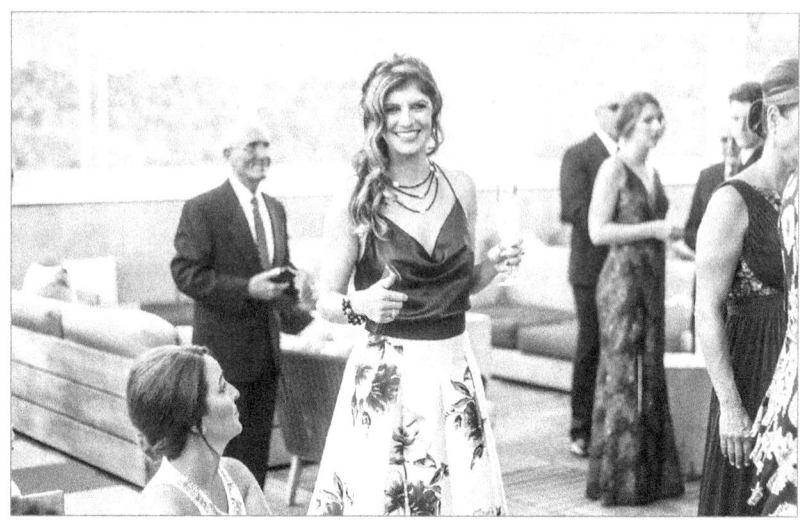

In 2018 Steven and I were married in Palm Springs. Since art played a major role in my career, we rented the Palm Springs Museum of Art. The wedding party began on the rooftop of our hotel, the Kimpton Rowan Palm Springs. Daniela, one of my project managers (for years) is in the center of this pic.

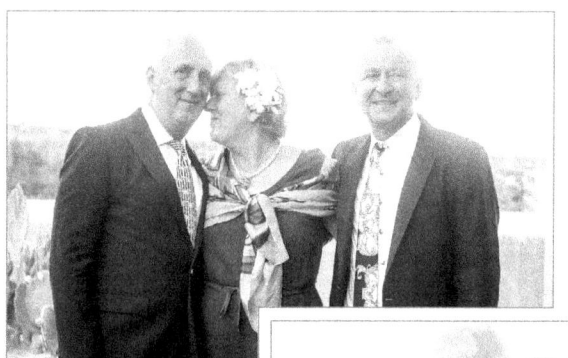

After spending so many years together, Susan Tjarksen became my "day" wife. She has a real husband to spend the nights with but we love her too.

We love Leslie too.
We love a lot of people.

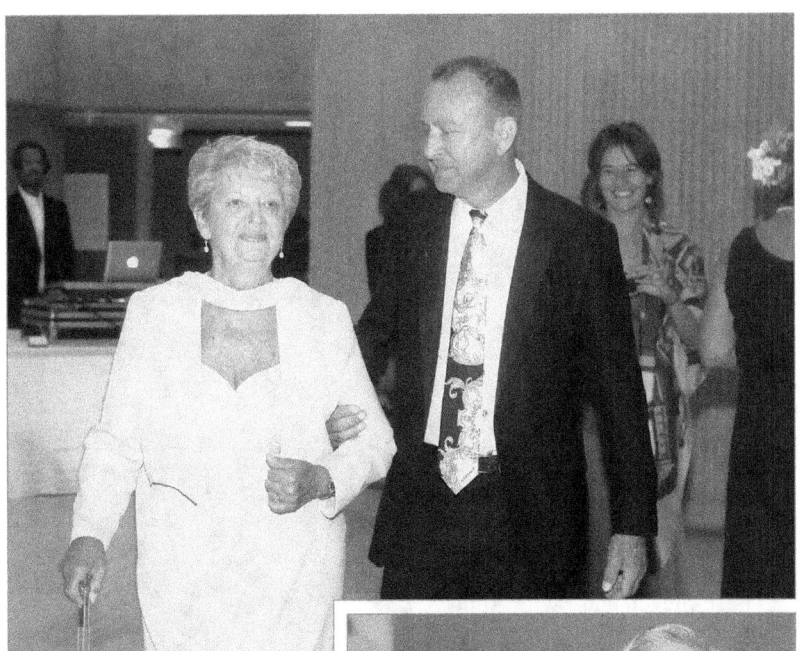

Mom gave me away. Not certain how these things work, she wasn't sure if she was supposed to pay for the wedding. We didn't know either so instead, she and Marty a.k.a. Daddy O hosted the rehearsal dinner.

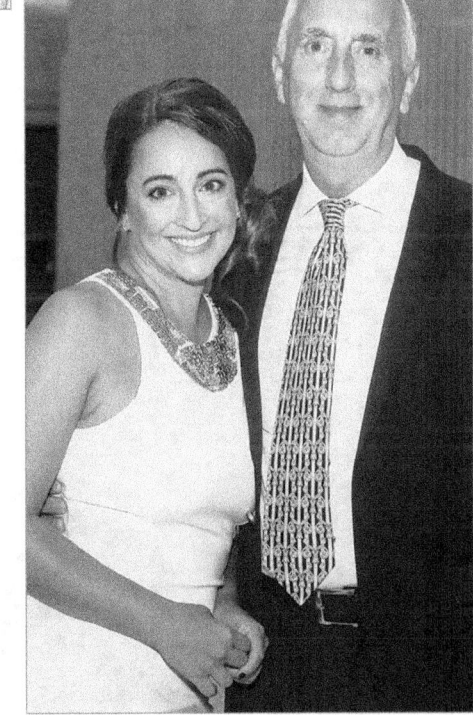

Jenna proudly gave away her father.

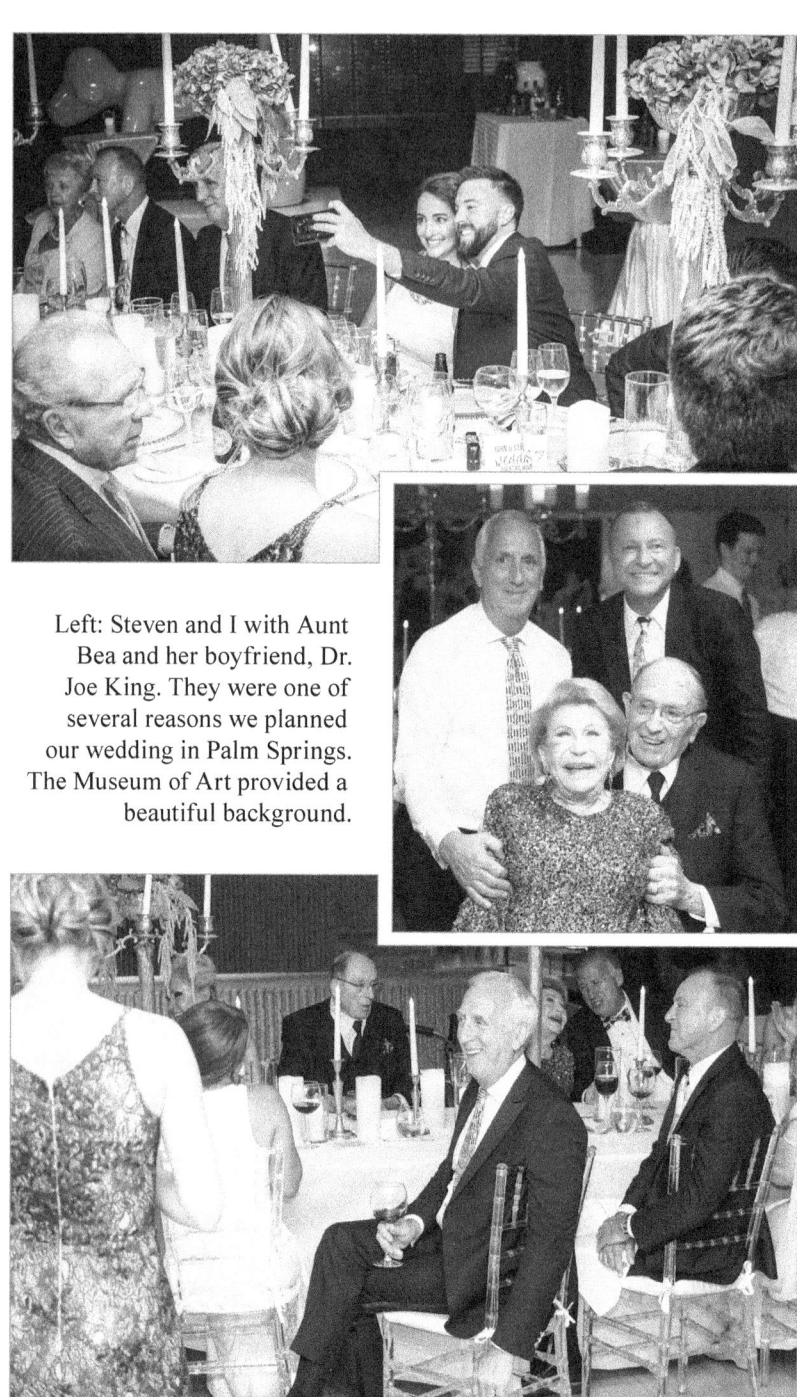

Left: Steven and I with Aunt Bea and her boyfriend, Dr. Joe King. They were one of several reasons we planned our wedding in Palm Springs. The Museum of Art provided a beautiful background.

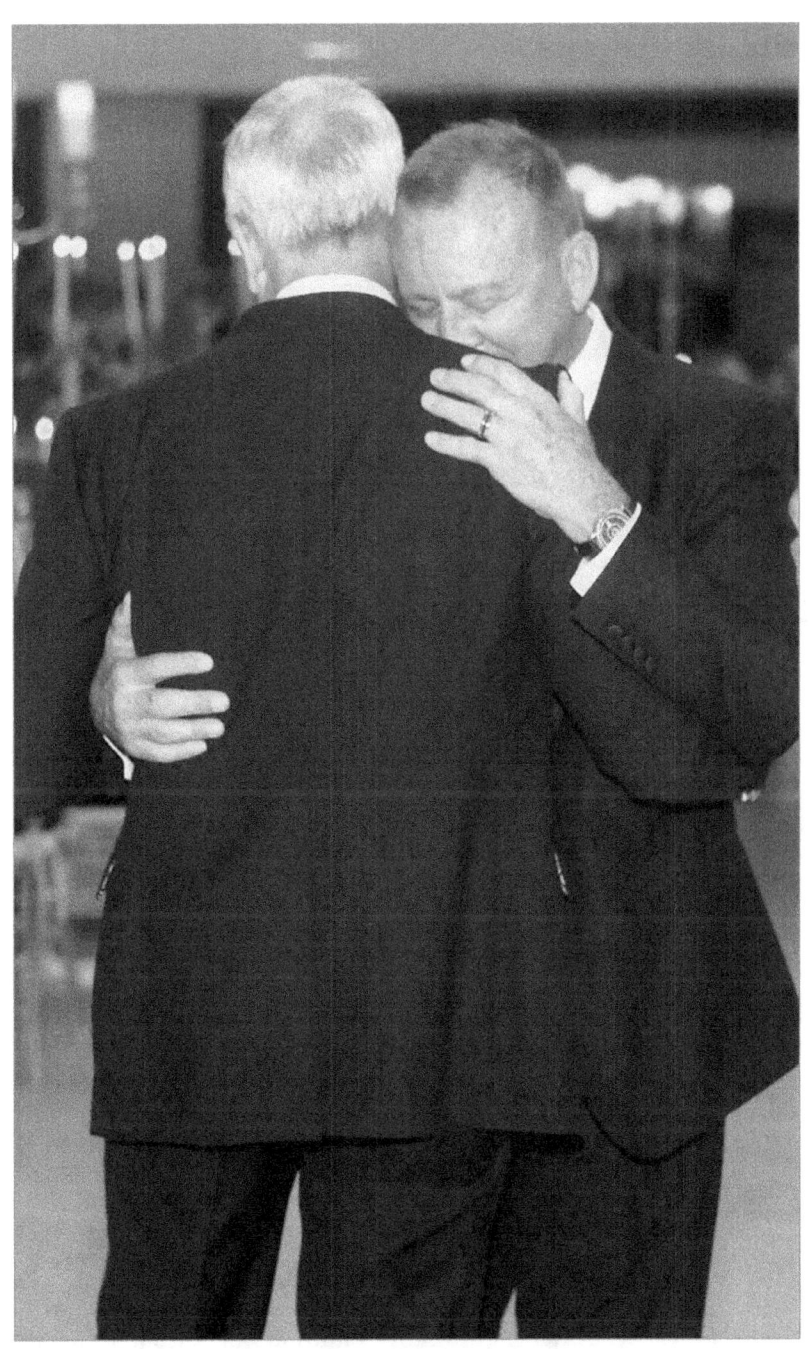

The happiest day of my life.

THE HOUSE THAT BUILT ME

After my parents re-divorced, Dad married a woman named Liz while at a carpet convention dinner. Since it was an industry event, we were not invited. Well, that's what he told us via post cards sent while the newlyweds honeymooned.

"Having a great time cruising the Caribbean. BTW. Got married. Love Dad and Liz."

I met Liz twice in my lifetime. The first occasion was the Christmas after they wed. They came to Chicago so Dad could introduce us to our stepmother. I was still so mad at him I gave Dad a lump of coal in a small velvet pouch. I bought her the Christian Dior fragrance "Poison."

Think they got the message?

The second time was at father's funeral. He died in a hotel room from an abdominal aortic aneurysm. This is most common in older men and smokers (he was both). He did this preceding the weekend Ray and Gail were supposed to get married. Whether he intentionally planned his demise this way no one knows. He couldn't tell us once he bled to death.

Mom thought it was her fault. For years she prayed to God to keep Dad away from her. She did not want him back in her life. And even though he was married—he still called her to say how much he missed her.

So, what happened? God answered Mom's prayers. Dad died and then she felt guilty. To sooth her we said it wasn't like she hired a hit man to do him in. For many more years she cried because she felt she killed Dad. In the meantime, a line had formed outside her condo door of people requesting special prayers from her. She has a direct line.

***

Working late one evening several months later, the phone rang. The caller said his realtor referred me because the house she sold him needed work. Ray Capitanini introduced himself saying he and his brother were owners of… I recognized his name and finished the sentence for him. I had been going to the *Italian Village Restaurant* since the Chagall mosaic was installed across the street.

When I met Ray and his Yugoslavian wife Nada, I had no idea he would become the father figure I never had. They were living in the top floor apartment of a three-flat near their new house. Its rooftop terrace was filled with plants. With no elevator, going home was a daily workout before workouts were fashionable. The roof leaked and at night, when it rained, they kept a bucket between them on the bed. They slept that way for years. What can I say? He was born under a water sign. Ray had an 18-year-old car he rarely drove because he took the elevated train to work. We talked for hours about his ideas for the architectural changes he wanted to make.

The realtor already installed her husband as general contractor and suggested an architect. I was the last man admitted to the team but the only one remaining on the job for almost twenty-five years. The general contractor, the architect and I were hired to gut the kitchen. Ray insisted it be restaurant quality. And they wanted a breakfast room, which meant an addition. Flooring and furniture were needed throughout.

We prepared drawings illustrating various design ideas for close to one year. Even though we provided renderings, Ray couldn't visualize the finished product. Finally, I convinced him to let us start. When the walls were framed he would begin to understand the architectural changes we proposed. If he didn't like it we could make changes however, it cost money to own the house and let it sit there. That bothered me.

Unfortunately, the contractor ripped Ray off for almost $250,000. He kept taking deposits for merchandise which never showed up. I heard of similar horror stories but never thought it would occur on one of my projects. WBBM-TV journalist Walter Jacobson aired an account about the scam artist embezzling money from Polish immigrants and our client. *Chicago Magazine* editorialized how the contractor lived the highlife off other people's money. His address was a prominent Lake Shore Drive high-rise and when no one was looking, he drove a Rolls Royce.

The architect's drawings included a nine-inch error in the interior width of the 25-foot-wide building and ultimately, after several other mistakes, Ray fired him. Alcohol later claimed the man's life.

By the time their "castello" was completed, Ray and Nada acquired their dream restaurant-quality kitchen and breakfast room. Heated floors were installed everywhere including the exterior terraces and sidewalks. Ray never again had to shovel the snow, but now in his 80's, he shovels for his elderly neighbors.

We excavated the basement to achieve a respectable ceiling height. It includes a paneled, critical listening room which doubles as Ray's office, a wine cellar, guest bedroom, full bath, bar and sitting area with an antique iron fireplace mantel.

I designed magnificent crotch-matched mahogany veneered doors with gold plated hinges and lever handles. The four bathrooms and powder room have gold or platinum sinks and faucets. Halfway into the construction a full third floor was added. It featured an outdoor terrace, exercise room, laundry room and another staircase concealed in a turret leading to the multi-level roof top with an outdoor shower, kitchen, assorted seating, plantings and Juliet balcony.

With varying levels, Ray needed an elevator to get his mother from point A to point D, E or F. That required another addition and modifications to the exterior design. The extra floors required new load calculations meaning we had to beef up the foundation to support the additional weight. These changes required engineers, time and more permits.

Then Ray said he and Nada did not want to gaze from the balconies at the rear of their house and see the air conditioning condensers on the roof of his garage. Therefore, a garden was created to conceal them. Copper planters, brick veneer, and a reflection pool that dropped three-hundred gallons of water per minute into a lily pond below needed steel I-beams to support the estimated twenty-thousand pounds. Ray, who is a modern-day Medici, embraced the idea.

The total renovation took seven years before my clients could move in. An iron walkway connected the garage rooftop to the second floor of their home after the building inspectors were gone.

On many occasions, Jeff and I were invited to dinner with Ray and Nada. (After his two-year hiatus Jeff moved back in with me.) We ate at the kitchen table as families often do. Their housekeeper prepared and served our meals. It was a very privileged time.

At the same time, Regina and I devoted many hours planning the 10th Annual BBF Auction. She was the undisputed queen of the ball. Her star-quality appearance captured the attention of photographers from all the city newspapers. Raising $150,000 net for the Better Boys Foundation, our first attempt at producing a charity event was deemed a rollicking success. And, as soon as the lights went out that night, we were immersed in planning auction #11.

We worked hard at making our affairs different from other fundraisers. After closing the silent auction and instructing our guests to take their seats we dimmed the lights in the grand ballroom and illuminated it with indoor fireworks. It was awesome. When the fireworks finished a spotlight focused on the podium where Regina and I stood and announced, in tandem, "Hi. We're back!"

A steel drum orchestra provided dinner music at the Better Boys Foundation's 11th event. A Jamaican limbo band performed dance music afterwards as women in strapless gowns sauntered beneath the bamboo pole.

Our live auction featured a racehorse. We did not drug him to cooperate—promise. I was afraid the horse would allow nature to take its course on stage, but—luckily—that did not happen. The $175,000 we raised that year helped fund numerous educational, counseling, and homeless youth programs.

"What will the Better Boys Foundation ever do to top what went on at this year's 11th annual Celebrity Auction?" observed *Chicago Sun-Times's* social columnist Mary Cameron Frye. We were both proud and humbled.

I donated my time and efforts to other needy organizations too. The *Landmark Preservation Council of Illinois;* a non-for-profit that tries to save architecturally and historically significant structures. The *Chicago Academy for the Arts,* an independent high school for the performing and visual arts named a National School of Distinction by the John F. Kennedy Center for the Performing Arts. It is the setting for the movie *Fame.* The *Chicago Film Festival,* the longest running competitive film festival in North America. The *Juvenile Diabetes Research Foundation* which funds type 1 diabetes research.

While battling the complications of Type 1 Diabetes and running a business full time, I tried to make time to give back to others. As Mahatma Gandhi once said, "the best way to find yourself is to lose yourself in the service of others."

COUNT YOUR
BLESSINGS

For some ungodly reason, my age—no matter what it was—continued to be an issue in my work life. That seemed behind me until, at thirty-one and three quarters, I was the youngest person to receive the Chicago Merchandise Mart's "Outstanding Achievement in the Interior Design Profession" award.

The previous year, 1990, my friend, Cal Ashford received the same honor. When I approached his table to offer congratulations Whitney Houston sat next to him. She, Diana Ross and Dionne Warwick were clients referred to him by his brother, Nick, and sister-in-law, Valerie Simpson of the legendary songwriting, singing duo, Ashford and Simpson.

That night Cal was dripping in gold and diamonds. Big ones. He was dressed in the most outrageous outfit from the ladies' department at Ultimo, a high-end Oak Street fashionista destination. He truly was the QUEEN of the Chicago design world.

Cal responded to my congratulations in loud clear sing-song tones heard by everyone around him "Don't worry dear, you'll receive the award next year."

Whether he really believed it or not, I thanked him wording "From your mouth to God's ears," and smiled at everyone at his table.

So when the letter arrived the following year from the Merchandise Mart informing me I was the recipient of the award, the first person I called, before Mom or Jeff, was Cal. I was in such shock my hands shook. I had to check my blood sugar to determine it wasn't low. It was hard to imagine my peers thought enough of me and my work to grant this distinction. I had plenty of stellar competition.

So many thoughts spun through my head. How did Cal know? Was he psychic? I was so choked up I could hardly talk. His response was the title of one of his brother and sister-in-law's songs...*Count Your Blessings.*

My family and friends totaled more than seventy guests at the Design Ball held in the Beaux Arts styled grand ballroom of the Conrad Hilton on Michigan Avenue. If traditional grandeur is your thing, this is one of the most elegant ballrooms in Chicago. Colossal arches gracefully reach towards the center of the multi chandeliered ceiling flanked by mirrors and crystal sconces. It was the perfect setting to honor Chicago's architecture and design talent.

Stepping up to the microphone in a black and white speckled Versace dinner jacket, I hoped I looked like the sophisticated trend setter I worked so hard to become. Wanting to sound like the consummate professional, I practiced my speech a million times. Spotlights came at me from every angle creating an intense glare in my one good eye. I worried I would not be able to read my cue cards.

Clients, vendors, friends, and, of course, my family were in attendance to witness the presentation. It was intimidating.

Acknowledging the fact that my work could only be as good as my clients allowed it to be I thanked them. Recognizing I could have the most creative ideas, but without the talented tradespeople needed to implement them, they had no value. I expressed gratitude to my vendors. I thanked my staff. Where would I be without them? Certainly not on the dais, so I accepted it as our award. Finally, I revealed to almost 800 people, some who knew me but more who did not, how my mother gave me a second chance at life when she gave me one of her kidneys. The spotlight moved to Mom. In tears, she rose from her chair followed by everyone in the room.

For years, I worried long and hard about people finding out about the extent of my illness. But that night, I took the opportunity to finally come out of the type 1 diabetes closet.

In June 1993 I received an even better honor. Mom came to work with me. She was tired of the long hours and corporate backstabbing at her car rental sales job. When she was working, I called her Jean not Mommy. We lunched together everyday spending quality time together for sixteen years. She sold potential customers on my philosophy of thinking outside the box while integrating art, architecture, and design delivering excellence and superior quality. She handled complaints. Sometimes she went to job sites to check on the work in progress.

And she signed checks which meant I could go away for a couple of weeks at a time. For years, she was the only other person in my office authorized to do so. Frank Barbaria had an accountant who signed his checks and embezzled over $100,000 from him, back in the '70's when that was real money. I learned from that robbery which is why no one else signed checks for me before Mom. I made her Secretary/Treasurer of JRWD. It was hard work and in the beginning, she was afraid she wasn't qualified.

"How did you learn to do all this?" she asked. But she did an excellent job, was the consummate ambassador and despite all the bull, we had a gas.

TWO AMERICANS
IN PARIS

I worked long hours thinking that would make up for my lack of education although the University of Hard Knocks provided me with numerous degrees. And I had my good luck charm. Mom. She was heaven sent and very smart which she credited to the nuns.

Since the transplant, my health was stable. The immuno-suppressants caused my blood pressure to rise but there were pills for that. I had a personal trainer who forced me to exercise. I was strong. I could run fast. And Jeff was home waiting for me at the end of the day.

Life was good.

After completing several model homes in Michigan Avenue's newest luxury high-rise, homeowners there and elsewhere began asking for help with their condos.

The death of her husband pushed Gertrude to sell her half floor co-op at the prestigious Drake Towers. After one showing a buyer paid a record full price for her 3,600 square foot residence planning to gut it. Why? Because they could.

She was devastated never imagining it would be snapped up so quickly.

We shopped for condos in every building up and down The Avenue but leaving the building that had been her home for 25 years proved too difficult. Gertrude selected another residence at the same address. And it was stunning. Two publications featured her new co-op before I completed it.

There was also a new venue in Chicago for architects and designers. Lofts. Contrary to the beliefs of many, loft living did not originate in New York City. No. It had been around long before. In fact, the most popular opera of all times, *La Boehme*, first performed in 1896, is set in a nineteenth century Parisian artist's loft.

In the fifties, artists starting renting space in commercial or industrial buildings in New York City for little money. The large primitive spaces, some without hot water, were perfect for starving artists. Years later that changed. In 2018, the most expensive loft in Lower Manhattan was marketed for $65-million dollars.

In the 90's, Chicago's loft condominium market had buyers standing in line. While working on several suburban McMansions and in Chicago's toniest buildings, I was also challenged to create homes made in former run-down factories with mega ceiling heights, abundant daylight, and raw finishes.

This is where I met two of my best friends, Susan and Bill. Both started out as clients, but our occupational enthusiasm made us inseparable.

Susan worked for a division of American Invsco, owned and operated by the Gouletas family—the Kardashians of the '80's.

Nicholas S. Gouletas was dubbed the "Condo King" of the 80s and 90s. His firm, American Invsco (AI), converted or built at least forty-five thousand condominiums around the country.

Evangeline Gouletas, Nick's sister and partner married New York Governor, Hugh Carey. She informed Governor Carey of a former marriage, claiming she was widowed—her daughter's father died. (That's what she told the daughter too.) After the wedding, the Governor discovered the "dead" husband opening a restaurant in Van Nuys, California. Two other ex-husbands were also uncovered. None of them six feet under. Her marriage to the governor ended in divorce.

Back then I yearned to champion AI as one of my clients. I wanted to design model homes, lobbies and the common areas for some of their buildings, but for years, the firm immediately across the hall from my office was their professional designer of choice. So in 1995, when Susan Tjarksen of American Invsco phoned my office, I was stunned. It seemed one of my dreams was about to come true. Finally, THEY were calling me. However, I was also scared. Rumor had it AI failed to pay their subcontractors and investors.

Susan was the project manager for *Haberdasher Square*, a conversion originally home to a menswear manufacturer. The building was converted to "loftominiums". Webster's does not recognize that word, but YOU try telling that to Nick Gouletas who was brilliant at marketing and the consummate salesperson. I learned a great deal from him.

My first loft model home was in a building on the Chicago River. It prompted Susan to hire me to design several models for her project. While visiting the upper floors of her development during construction, I passed out from low blood sugar. Really low. My head was spinning like a top. The foreman picked me up, carried me into the construction elevator and put me down in Susan's office.

Scared the shit out of everyone.

I met Bill Senne in his Bucktown neighborhood restaurant *Jane's*. It was a few blocks away from the latest building I purchased and remodeled converting 6 apartments into 3 larger ones. I was still playing with the idea of being a real estate developer as I worked with, and learned from, so many of them.

Jeff and I dined at Jane's often. It was close by and we loved their food. One-night Jane (Bill) approached our table asking if I was the "famous" interior designer John Robert Wiltgen. He actually used the word "famous". I looked around to make sure he meant me. Bill's real estate sales firm was marketing a loft development and he wanted JRWD to create the model. It was the first of many buildings I worked on with him. I also designed three beautiful homes for him and his family to live in. They were all featured in numerous magazines.

***

Not having had a real vacation for several years, I decided Jeff and I would go to Europe. But not without many debates with his mother.

"You're not taking my son 4,000 miles away from home," she ordered on the phone.

"Rose, your son is thirty-six. I think he's finally old enough to make up his own mind. Eighty-four thousand, one hundred people from the US fly to Europe every day—not counting the pilots and flight attendants."

"You think you're so smart. You're not afraid of shit…" Those were her exact words. Truth is, I'm afraid of a lot of shit, but I refuse to let my fears stop me from enjoying life. I wanted to tell her that, but she hung up before giving me the chance.

We were going to Paris via Brussels. I wanted to see my friends, Kurt and Lara. She is and always will be one of the great loves of my life. We were friends and dance partners during the disco days while Leana was away at school and before, during and after Rhonda. Lara was eighteen when we met. I was going on seventeen. Neither one of us were old enough to go to Faces but I had a membership and platinum American Express card, AND she always looked stunning—so our entry was not denied.

A photo from her modeling composite of her laying naked on a beach wrapped in seaweed was flashed up on this huge screen for everyone to see when she and I were on the dance floor. She has been my friend longer than almost anyone else and I am fortunate we are still connected.

Lara met her husband in Kuwait when she and her older sister, Anna, hosted a fashion show for a handful of sheiks and sultans each having more wives than they could count. Anna designed and manufactured extravagant clothing in Bangkok, where she lived on a python farm. Kurt was the general manager of the SAS Hotel in Kuwait. It was there they met and fell in love. Within a short time, they married and ultimately ended up in Oslo, where I spent time with them when AJ and I went to see King Olav V.

This was Jeff's first trip to Europe and as we traveled across the pond he was plenty nervous. In fact, he never traveled that far ever again. He loathed sitting on a plane for nine plus hours, even in Business Class. I always thought of it as the prelude to another adventure.

When the captain announced it was time to land Jeff asked where we were meeting Lara.

"I don't know," I replied. That was the truth. I didn't have the foggiest.

He exploded "What do you mean you don't know?"

Nearby passengers looked our way.

"Jeff," I responded in an exaggerated whisper. "I've never been to this airport, so if she told me to meet her at My Little Cup Coffee Spot in the international terminal, I wouldn't have a clue where to go. Would you?"

"You are crazy," People were still staring. "I should have listened to my mother and stayed home."

After we exited the aircraft, gathered our luggage (seven pieces between us) and cleared customs we were in a sea of Belgian residents, businesspeople and tourists. Jeff looked at me and rather sarcastically asked, "Well, now what?"

I didn't say a word. I just nodded my head slightly forward. It was like the story in the Bible about Moses parting the sea.

The crowd split with some going left and others to the right. Thirty meters ahead stood a vision. Blonde hair. Beautiful, full red lips. Big, black sunglasses. Gold chunky earrings. A top with an actual gold chained collar printed with Renaissance paintings. Perfectly fitted blue jeans with a big chunky belt. She looked as if she just walked off the runway.

"Is that her?"

"What do you think?" I answered dropping my bags to run to her.

Kurt and Lara lived in an exquisite Art Deco palace that was subdivided into several homes. Decorated with bright colored Thai silks it was totally unexpected in this conservative city housing NATO headquarters. Tall ceilings and an antique crystal chandelier suspended over a buffed and polished piano. A long red silk sofa in the living room beneath two Tibetan tapestries. Lots of vividly lacquered Orientalia mixed with majestic Empire furniture.

Two floor-to-ceiling doors between the dining room and kitchen opened automatically when approached. The state-of-the-art kitchen was complete with a handsome young chef. We drank lots of sweet champagne, dined at one of Kurt's *Michelin* star restaurants, stayed overnight in one of their beautiful guest rooms and after breakfast, caught the train to Paris.

This was the first Parisian excursion for both of us. Other than *bon jour, merci* and *escargot* neither of us spoke the language. We walked a lot. Sometimes took the metro. I loved the stations decorated with remarkable sculptures and other works of art. The Garnier Opera House with its seven-ton chandelier— the setting for Andrew Lloyd Weber's play *Phantom of the Opera*—was perfection. I spent hours admiring the intricately patterned marble floors and mosaic ceiling by Marc Chagall and wondered what secrets hid behind the locked French polished doors. Discovering the magnificent courtyard of the Palais Royale with its colorful garden, fountains and modern Daniel Buren sculpture made me imagine the life of Louis XIV when he lived there as a child. Versailles. Oh my God. Standing at the gold-plated entrance gates, tears ran down my face. What one could do with a hunting lodge and a few scheckles! I was overwhelmed and didn't know where to look first. There was so much to see, so much detail. The thought of all the drawings, prepared by hand, required to build such an exquisite palace was overwhelming.

Every morning or at the end of every evening Jeff switched on the tele to watch his latest discovery—Euro VH1. He was enamored with artists he'd never seen before. The Army of Lovers—a Swedish dance music group (originally hair-dressers)—became his latest obsession. After that I spent a day at the Louvre as he visited Virgin Records. I visited the Musee d'Orsay, the train station converted into a museum, while he returned to the music store.

Soon it was time to go home but I'd be back.

I knew the vacation was over when, during an unscheduled visit, Dr. Oyer insisted on rushing me to the hospital. He was always rushing me there. Why couldn't we take our time?

The second toe of my right foot was swollen from cellulitis. A red line (blood poisoning) was inching its way up my leg. Dr. Giegerich prescribed an IV antibiotic to treat the infection and while he thought I had a good chance to heal, there was a possibility a pocket of pus could lead to amputation—even death.

Why do doctors do that? Terrify their patients?

Of course, I was afraid. Again. But I wasn't going to die no matter what the doctor said. It had been exactly 10 years since acute thigh pain blamed on cellulitis first introduced me to Dr. Giegerich. Now the real battle began.

In an operating room Giegerich made an incision over the bone of the second toe exposing the degenerated site. A build-up of infected fluid was partially responsible for the swelling. I was overwhelmed at the thought of amputation—even though it was just a toe. Having spent so many years trying to make people's worlds beautiful now I might become unattractive.

Everyone tried to cheer me up.

"It's only a toe."

"You'll hide it in your shoe."

"No one is going to know it's gone."

But they couldn't relieve my anxiety. And let's be clear, it is only a toe when it is someone else's foot.

Fortunately, Giegerich did not have to remove it. The next day, in another operating room, a PICC line (Peripherally Inserted Central Catheter) was put into my arm so I could infuse IV antibiotics myself. The long plastic tube went all the way to my heart and stayed there for 3 months. Night and day, every day, for 90 days, I connected the PICC line to an elastomeric pump containing the antibiotics.

Silently I prayed thinking someone other than those wearing white lab coats might need to save me. You never know when you are going to need God. I learned He does come in handy every now and then.

LIVIN' LA VIDA LOCA

In my mid 30's, I was working on an all-encompassing project in Rancho Santa Fe, California deemed one of the best places to live in Southern Cal. I recently finished a Michigan Avenue condominium for these clients which was featured in the *New York Times Sunday Magazine* and on HGTV. Therefore, they expected the same of me for their west coast home.

He was one of the financial experts behind Reaganomics but requested my help in deciding which southern California property to purchase. She was young enough to be his daughter and looked like Nicole Kidman when she starred in the movie *Dead Calm*. Before asking me to join them, they narrowed their choice of houses to three. I suggested making an offer on the least expensive. No matter which home they acquired it would be gutted and renovated. Therefore, the least expensive option, a 5,000-square foot ranch on five-acres, still costing millions would enable them to do everything we dreamed of and more. What would my client offer the sellers? He told me the round number he was thinking of. I suggested he reduce the sum by $25,000.00. He asked why.

This was my answer: "When you and Karen married, you went to City Hall. She never received a ring. With the $25,000.00, I could take her to a wholesale jeweler I know and get a lovely rock in a gorgeous setting."

She loved that idea! Their realtor wrote the offer according to my recommendation. It was accepted, and the wife treasured their new home even more. There are all sorts of ways to make your clients happy.

On completion, their slump block and glass ranch house was transformed into an elegant 11,000-square foot retreat not including the freestanding guest house. For two people. It included the largest master bath I ever designed featuring separate rooms for his and her toilets. His included bookshelves and a TV. The two person Whirlpool tub was set against a large glass window flanked by sliding doors which lead to a private garden in which they played "chase me" dressed as Adam and Eve. There was a party sized jetted tub too—the more the merrier. Open the doors to a lush landscape with specimen trees and a massive Fernando Botero sculpture originally part of an exhibit in Chicago's Grant Park.

Newsweek took notice. In a feature on luxurious baths, I received top billing over internationally acclaimed designer Phillipe Starke which was a huge ego booster FOR ME. My bathroom creation also received an international design award.

While working on this residence I discovered the opulent Beverly Hills Hotel often referred to as the Pink Palace. I was constantly driving up the 405 to LA—its resources for the house were endless. On one trip, I decided to take Mom with so she could see the estate. We asked Gertrude to join us. She was a faithful patron of the five-star Beverly Hills Hotel and Bungalows for more years than I was old, and suggested we stay there several nights before driving south to Rancho Santa Fe. The minute we pulled up the palm tree lined drive to the Bruce Wayne looking valet, who greeted us under a green and white striped awning, I knew we were not in Kansas.

The hotel had been closed two-and-a-half years for a $100 million-dollar plus renovation. The finished design was magic.

We walked up the red carpet which led to the art deco lobby. Gold leaf, pink and green with accents of persimmon. Dramatic but elegant and refined. It looked expensive and it was. It's so true, if you had to ask you couldn't afford it, so Mom and I shared a room on the ground floor with a private landscaped terrace. It was decorated in more of the same shades of peachy-pink and green. The glamorous marble bathroom was thoughtfully detailed in similar colored marbles and its window shade was motorized. In the 90's.

Mom felt like a Queen and me—a Prince. After that I was hooked and stayed at the legendary property often. Concealed behind palm trees, banana leaves and exotic flowers it was my entre to a world of A-lister film stars and celebrities.

NOBODY WALKS
IN LA

Sometimes we meet someone with whom there is an instant connection—as if we've known them forever. Perhaps in a past life. When I've encountered a person I knew centuries ago, the connection feels deeper than with friends I made for the first time. I met numerous people I felt that way about—and, hopefully, they about me. Jeff is an old soul and was my brother two hundred years ago.

It was love at first sight for "Miss Hollywood" and moi. I coined that nickname for her because she was friendly with members of the "Brat Pack", and she was the one who introduced me to the sparkle of Tinsel Town.

It all began one day back in 1996 as I sat at my desk. Mom said I received a call from a Karen Murphy with Dyansen Art Gallery on Rodeo Drive. Jean (it was office hours) suspected she was a solicitor. I was intrigued by the fact she was from Beverly Hills and picked up line two.

"Is this John?" asked a friendly voice.

"It is."

"Hi John. I'm Karen Murphy calling from Dyansen Galleries on Rodeo Drive. You were here a few weeks ago, but I was out so we didn't get a chance to meet. We are having a private, invitation only dinner this Thursday for Alexandra Nichita, a Romanian cubist artist we discovered, followed by the public opening of our show for her on Friday. She is ten years old and already in the most impressive collections. Oprah owns one of her paintings. So do Lee Iacocca and David Geffen. We call her the 10-year-old Picasso. You'll understand when you see her work. I'm calling to personally invite you to be my guest. It's an intimate affair. There will only be 50 people total, including the heads of Walt Disney, Sony, the artist, and her parents."

"Let me check my calendar," I replied gazing out the windows of my corner office as I spun around in my black leather executive chair. Immediately I decided I was going. When my chair stopped, I continued. "This is a busy week for me however I will have one of my assistants move some things around. What time?"

"6:00."

"Perfect. Karen, thank you for calling. I look forward to meeting you."

I used American Airlines miles for a free ticket to LA. I was going to be one of 50 people at a private party on Rodeo Drive that, in the end, cost me $65,000 plus whatever I paid for three nights at the Beverly Hills Hotel. In retrospect, it would have been much cheaper to buy the airplane ticket—not the painting.

When I met Karen, I was in love. L O V E. We never met but somehow, she recognized me in the pre-Facebook days as I checked in with security at the door. After a hug and kiss-kiss this blonde bombshell *a la* Veronica Lake whisked me off to preview the exhibit. In very high heels she wore a very fitted ivory, somewhat lowcut dress that nicely showed off her… legs. We walked arm in arm, stopping methodically, to discuss each painting.

Alexandra was talented. The geometric angles and shapes of her two-dimensional paintings were bold explosions of color. Expressive. Each included a brief story of its inspiration. Several had red stickers on the wall next to them indicating they were sold. I didn't want to miss my chance to acquire one. The painting I purchased spoke to me. It has all the same colors of my logo—which I love. Mustard. Olive Green. Tomato. Black.

The little girl is going places I thought. So am I.

I loved Beverly Hills. Rodeo Drive. The Pink Palace. For years I hosted an annual, some years, semi-annual "pool party" at the hotel and invited clients and friends—some who Karen introduced me to.

After the opening of Alexandra's show, Karen asked me to dinner. In a sexy vintage Jaguar, she drove us to her favorite spot in Brentwood. The maître d' smiled at Karen and led us to a red leather booth where she introduced me to her husband, Bobby Cooper, an actor. She proudly acknowledged he recently completed a Nick Cassavetes film, *Unhook the Stars*, with Gena Rowlands, Marisa Tomei and Gerard Depardieu. The previous year, he appeared in *The Crossing Guard* directed by Sean Penn.

Bobby got up and shook my hand as Karen slid into the booth sitting between us. She then told Bobby about me. How she knew the things she said was baffling. In 1996 only 10-million people used the internet maybe once a month. Today more than three billion are online every day. No Google, Wikipedia or Facebook then. Over dinner Bobby told me about a film he was currently working on, *She's So Lovely,* starring Sean Penn, Robin Wright, and John Travolta.

It was so exciting. I didn't want to leave Beverly Hills.

In one weekend, I made some great friends and began dreaming about designing homes for LA's rich and famous. Karen asked me to stay in touch—which I did. At home I tried to sell Alexandra Nichita paintings and prints to all my clients just so I could speak with her. Even Jean bought one which she still has and loves.

Afterwards I found every possible excuse to go to LA. It was not always the best thing for my diabetes. Fresh baked cookies were left on the bedside table of my hotel room at night. And I ate out every meal. But it was great for me mentally. I was living my life better than I ever dreamed and loving every minute of it.

One evening Karen, Bobby and I attended the premier of a play starring Sean Penn's Mom and Dad with James Gandolfini of *The Soprano's* fame. Afterwards, Sean invited us to the cast party. Karen seated me next to Robin Wright Penn. Well, maybe forced me. Otherwise I wouldn't have. Outside my own controlled environments, I can be noticeably shy, but Robin was nice. Engaging. I asked her about their kids and the carjacking in their Santa Monica driveway. It was already old news, but I was interested in hearing her version. Robin demanded the criminal's hand over her children before giving them the keys to her Toyota. Robin and I spoke for some time. But there were others who also wanted their fifteen minutes of fame with *The Princess Bride* and Jenny from *Forest Gump*. And they all wondered who I was in my Versace suit with buttonholes EVERYWHERE.

Another time, Jeff and I attended the cast party for *Message in a Bottle* starring Robin and Kevin Costner. When the party was over, we were invited back to Sean and Robin's Four Seasons hotel suite. The following day we had lunch with them at a cafe on Cannon Drive. I felt bad for the Hollywood power couple. People kept coming up to them asking for autographs or complimenting them on their films. After a while, Bobby took control and ushered fans away from our table so Sean could finally take a bite of his sandwich. Fame comes with a lot of perks but also a loss of privacy. Nonetheless, I would like to try it!

In Chicago, John Travolta was being honored with a Lifetime Achievement Award. I was on the Board of Directors of The Chicago International Film Festival and expected to buy a table at the annual gala. Bobby and Miss Hollywood came to Chicago and stayed with Jeff and me over the weekend. To impress them I spent a prince's ransom on new bedding for the master bedroom which they were going to use. Jeff and I stayed in the guest room.

As we were walking through the hotel lobby Bobby spotted Travolta. A group of FBI-look-a-likes were ushering him into a secure space so he could finish putting on his makeup. It looked like he started as he flew his own plane to the Windy City. Bobby ran through the band of security guards. John was surprised to see him.

"Coop, what are you doing here?" Travolta asked.

"Are you kidding?" Bobby replied. "I wouldn't have missed this." He waived us over. "These are my friends. This other John…," he pointed at me, "is on the board of directors for the Film Festival".

Miss Hollywood whipped a camera out of her handbag to snap a photo.

"You don't mind, do you John?" she flashed him a BIG smile.

"No, Murph, not at all." John moved in—his hand held tight somewhere lower than my back. There was no "Me Too" group for men back then. Not that it mattered. I took it as a compliment. I still have that photo framed. Karen blew it up bigger than life and gave it to me. It has moved with me three times.

Travolta was at the podium when Bobby ran to the stage almost knocking over one of the waiters. John was speaking as Bobby dialed Sean Penn on one of my other guest's cellphone. He wanted to say "hello" and "congratulations" to John. Travolta's security detail tried to stop him, but Bobby plowed his way through them.

Everyone in the audience was in shock. What was this crazy person doing? But when John explained Sean Penn was on his friend's cell phone, everyone applauded.

It was the craziest 5 minutes in Chicago Film Festival gala history.

Academy Award winning actor, Tim Hutton (*Ordinary People*), received an award from the Chicago International Children's Festival for his directorial debut of *Digging to China.* The story features the friendship between a pre-teen girl and an intellectually challenged adult male. Karen, Bobby,

Jeff, and I rooted for Tim when he came on stage. Karen took lots of pics.

Afterward several of us went to the home of one of my clients with a Miro print and Tim. I had been trying to get this couple to purchase some real artwork and having Tim Hutton along couldn't hurt. As we drove through assorted Chicago neighborhoods, he hung out the window of my car waving to young, college-age girls on the street. Some recognized him and did an exasperated double take.

"Was that really Tim Hutton?"

Tim carried the framed artwork and rang the bell while we hid. When the client, a doctor, opened the door I thought she would bust a gut.

How do you say that in medical lingo?

Amelia, the client, did a double take, closed the door in Tim's face and then opened it again to make sure he wasn't a hallucination. When we jumped out yelling "surprise," she knew he was for real. I provided unexpected craziness for my clients. Designing a home can be a royal pain in the ass. I tried to make the process fun and memorable for my customers.

We were invited into the family room where her husband was watching TV. She nonchalantly said, "Look honey, Tim Hutton's here." He was equally surprised and jumped up off the sofa to shake Tim's hand. Then everyone sat down to watch a college football game which lasted hours. Bobby was Tim's bookie. He was the bookie to half of Hollywood and there were lots of bets on this Ivy League battle.

When the game ended, Tim signaled time to go. Bobby looked awful. He lost a lot of money watching college football. I invited everyone to the Italian Village.

Sundays are for carbs and lots of them. After we devoured our authentic northern Italian dishes, we played poker in our private booth until after closing. The waiters kept bringing bottles of an expensive red wine Tim was particularly fond of, so much so that when he returned to Chicago once, he revisited the restaurant for the vino.

Bobbie helped me acquire two tickets to the 71st Academy Awards belonging to an A-List Actor. Not only was Bobbie a bookie and bit-part-actor, but he was also a scalper. They were twelfth row, main floor, center seats—my Christmas gift to Mom. I could never repay her for the kidney and all she's done to help me. Of course, we were staying at the Beverly Hills Hotel.

The Saturday evening before the Sunday awards show, Jeff and I took Mommy, Bobby, A.J., producers Peter and Bobby Farrelly, Timothy Hutton, and his girlfriend du jour to dinner at Spago—Wolfgang Puck's V.I.P. popular Beverly Hills restaurant. My star-studded entourage earned us the round table in the center of the courtyard. Without asking. Other celebrities, like Tony Curtis with some young thing who also sat outside, kept giving us the eye.

Tim and his date made out like crazy. There was no talking to them. When they finally came up for air, Mom reached across the table to shake the young lady's hand.

"I'm sorry dear, I didn't get your name..."

The table chatter ceased.

The date looked around the table. With the biggest smile I've ever seen she stood and reached back across the large table to shake Mommy's hand and replied, "Hi. My name's Angie." Tim had met her on the set of *Playing God*.

As Mom sat down, I whispered Angelina Jolie just won a Golden Globe Award for her role in *Gia*. Mommy's turn to be shocked, "Jesus. Joseph. And Mary," she gasped. Everyone broke out in laughter.

Angie noticed Jeff's tattooed arms peeking from his long-sleeved shirt. "You have tattoos?"

He nodded—like twenty times.

"Can I see them?" she asked.

"You want to see them?" he had to make sure.

She nodded.

He undid his cufflinks and rolled up his sleeves.

"Oh, they're amazing," she remarked.

"You like them?" he asked. Was she just being nice?

"Yes."

"Well, my whole back is done..."

Uh oh. Here we go.

"Really? Let me see." And with that she had him stand and helped him undo his shirt. The highlight of his life. He pulled it over his shoulders, so she could examine the painting on his back. When finished, she yanked his shirt down. He tried tucking it in.

"I have a tattoo," she admitted.

"You do?" Jeff was thrilled to share his love of this ancient art of inserting color and design beneath live human skin.

She nodded, smiling. Was she toying with him?

"Do you want to see it?"

"Yes." He was so excited.

She undid her pants revealing a tattoo in that private region most people never get to see in public. It was a Latin inscription

"Quod me nutrit me destuit," which she translated. "It means…
what nourishes me, destroys me."

The following morning Jeff did something very glam with
Mom's hair making her look like a Hollywood legend. If we
couldn't have a doctor in the family, might as well have a
hairdresser.

The hose from my PICC-line kept creeping out the cuff of my
shirt so Jeff cut the toes off one of my gym socks, wrapped the
hose around my upper arm and covered it with the sock. I was
very self-conscious of my PICC-line showing no matter where
I went.

When Mom and I arrived at the Dorothy Chandler Pavilion,
Sophia Loren exited her limo in front of ours. That's when it
became real for us. Mom and I were going to the Academy
Awards.

All of Hollywood royalty must clear security before they get
to the red carpet. It's like going through airport security if the
airport was in a tent. Mom was so nervous. We weren't supposed
to be there. The tickets clearly stated if you were not a member
of the Motion Picture Academy of Arts and Sciences you would
be considered trespassing and removed from the premises.

Walking through the metal detector the alarm went off. A
guard asked for her handbag. Mom's Altoids in their metal
strongbox were the culprit. With a lot of people starring, we
were quickly ushered out of the tent.

Mom and I put on our sunglasses and started to wave.

We were behind Ellen DeGeneres and Anne Heche. None
of the TV anchors wanted to interview us, so we kept waiving
until we breezed into the pre-Academy Awards cocktail party.

For her third time, Whoopee Goldberg was the hostess with the most costume changes of any Academy Awards show. She opened in "white face" dressed as Queen Elizabeth (the movie was nominated for 7 awards). The comedian-actress-producer introduced herself as the "African Queen" saying, "Some of you may know me as the Virgin Queen, but I can't imagine who."

In 1994 Whoopee went down in history for being the first-ever solo female host for the Oscar's. In 1999 she was brilliant again making the night fantastic—one of the best in Academy Awards history.

Italian actor Roberto Benigni won Best Actor for his role in *Life is Beautiful*. He literally crawled over the people in the rows in front of him to get to the stage. Despite much controversy and a bunch of protesters outside, the 89-year-old Elia Kazan received a lifetime achievement award. (In 1952 he named eight actors to the Congressional investigation of Communist infiltration in the entertainment industry.) Harvey Weinstein stole the microphone from Edward Zwick when they were on stage for producing Best Picture *Shakespeare in Love*. Years later, if you ask Mom about her night there, she still gets choked up and teary eyed.

The following morning Bobby called. He had to see me. Alone. Still half asleep I suggested the Polo Lounge in one hour. I connected the PICC line to my IV antibiotic, dressed and ran down the hallway to the iconic restaurant referred to as the Hollywood commissary.

The actress pretty hostess addressed me by name and said my guest had been seated. She escorted me to the table.

Bobby sat at the floor-to-ceiling plate glass window with a view of the huge Brazilian pepper tree growing in the walled-courtyard for almost a century. Outside, beneath the tree, is one of Mom's favorite spots at the hotel. There and the gardens surrounding the pool.

He looked awful. I sat down.

He asked how Mom liked the Academy Awards. I told him everything. Then he asked me for $10,000.00. I spit my Diet Coke out all over the white tablecloth.

"What do you need $10,000.00 for?" I choked. I just gave him $8,000.00 for the two tickets.

"John, you cannot tell Karen." Okay, first clue I thought. "But I am sick. I think I have colon cancer and need to have some tests. I don't have the money."

"What makes you think you have colon cancer?" I asked.

Did I really want to know?

He gave me the gory details, which no one should discuss over breakfast.

This did not seem like the typical conversation had by Hollywood deal makers. Or was it? No matter, I didn't believe him and wasn't going to give Bobby the money.

"I don't have the money..." I started.

"John, I have no place else to go," he pleaded.

How was that possible? He knew everyone in Hollywood.

Raising his voice caught the attention of other diners. "If I don't get these tests, I might die..."

"I'd like to help you. I would,"

"I'll pay you back. You know I will. Here look..." he pulled something from his jacket pocket. A long, blue velvet box with

FRED in gold letters spanning the center of the iconic container from world-renowned jeweler Fred Samuel. He opened it.

"This is the Patek Phillippe watch Charlie (Sheen) gave me for taking Brittany Ashland to the hospital after he grabbed her by the hair and slammed her onto the marble floor of his house. She split her lip. There was blood everywhere. Charlie was fucked up and said he was going to get some fishing line to sew her up. I calmed him down. Told him to take it easy and drove her to Cedars Sinai Medical Center." Where, I later learned, he barely stopped and told her to "Get out!" before taking off.

"What?"

"It's true," he said. "Charlie pled no contest in a suit filed by attorney Gloria Allred. A settlement was reached, and he got two years' probation. Here try it on." He took the watch from the box and handed it to me. "I want you to take the watch as collateral. When I finish paying you, you give me back the watch."

"Bobby, the only way I can make this work is if I get a cash advance on my credit card. BUT. It will come with twenty-one percent interest." Surely, he wouldn't agree to that.

He could borrow the money from a loan shark for less.

"Whatever you think is fair," he agreed. Christ. We finished our breakfast. I took the watch and told him I would get the money once I got home. And although I'd come to regret it because he never paid me back, I sent him a check. He didn't have cancer. He wasn't even bleeding from his you know what.

Years later when Miss Hollywood finally divorced him and I told her the story she said he probably owed his bookmaker money. He *was* a good actor.

***

I was constantly trying to get my foot in the door of the lifestyles of the rich and famous. Beverly Hills. Bel Air. Brentwood. Malibu. I wanted to provide my design services to someone/ anyone who owned a house in one of those areas. I kept going back and forth trying to look as if I lived there.

From my very large, elegant suite at the Beverly Hills Hotel I phoned Miss Hollywood suggesting she invite anyone and everyone to my next party. Friends from Chicago also flew to LA to attend my "Thank God Columbus Discovered America" get-together. I hired a comedic songstress and pianist for entertainment and served hors d'oeuvres shaped like the Nina, Pinta, and Santa Maria.

A couple of hours before the guests were expected the phone rang.

"John?" it sounded like a valley girl.

"Yes."

"Hi," more lively. "It's Jen..." Jennifer Nicholson. Jack's daughter. Also an actress known for her roles in *Jason Lives: Friday the 13th Part VI* and *The Witches of Eastwick*.

"Jen, how are you?" This was great. She called me.

"Hey, Mark (her husband) and I are excited about your party tonight. Would it be Okay if I brought a guest with us?"

"Oh my gosh, Jen, you could bring a bus load if you want."

"Thank you." Then in a whisper, "Someone is staying with us. My Dad said she might be my sister and, well, I don't know what to do with her..."

"Whether or not she is your sister, she is welcome. Come on down," sounding like a game show host. Honey Duffy, then eighteen, did turn out to be Jennifer's Danish half-sister and, in later years, Jack's favorite daughter.

Elaine Young, real estate agent to the stars including Elvis Presley, Elizabeth Taylor, Sonny and Cher came with her entourage. That was a big score for me. I hoped she would refer a client needing a professional designer.

Luckily she was the fourth wife of film star Gig Young, the father of her daughter Jennifer, who was roommates with former American madame Heidi Fleiss. Gig turned out to be a murderer shooting his fifth wife Kim Schmidt and then himself, three weeks after they married.

Elaine drove a Rolls Royce convertible to shuttle clients to some of Beverly Hills priciest properties. I left my laptop casually open during the party to a slideshow of my work so she could glimpse some of my completed projects. However, I removed my ad for "Bathrooms to Die For."

Georgia, a friend of mine from Chicago was staying with me. She caught my attention in the suite's kitchen as we refilled appetizer trays.

"John, it is snowing out there," she sounded like a spy.

I stared at her. "Georgia what are you talking about? It's 75-degrees. How could it be snowing?"

"No John, I mean it's *snowing...*" with one finger she covered a nostril.

"Oh my God," sticking my head out from the kitchen I peered into the gigantic living room. "Are you kidding me?"

"No. Just thought you should know," she said quietly.

I was petrified. What was I supposed to do with that bit of information? Go around and look up everyone's nose?

I didn't want to be arrested or tossed from the hotel.

I did exactly what the lead character in the Netflix series *The Crown* does. NOTHING. If anything happened, I would plead ignorance.

To say the least it was a wild evening. People were on the terrace, which wrapped around two sides of the hotel, throwing oranges at the windows of the suites above. These were adults.

The next morning I tiptoed into the living room. Suite 100 (later converted to a bar) looked as if a rock star partied all night. People were asleep everywhere. In no condition to drive home, they crashed on sofas, ottomans, the terrace, and piano bench.

It was 8 am. Georgia peeked from beneath her blanket and asked "does the word 'disaster' mean anything to you?"

Danny, a former Marine, slept on the floor next to her sofa with good intentions. Protect her no matter what. I was sure hotel management would never let me return.

Looking like Zombies, my blind friend Chris and I stumbled to the Polo Lounge for breakfast. I needed to eat. We sat at a table in the garden beneath the huge Pepper tree which is gone now, much to many guests' chagrin—including mine.

When we returned to our digs, the cast of characters were still asleep. Chris suggested we drive to the Buddhist Self Realization Fellowship Lake Shrine in Santa Monica. As we waited for the parking attendant to retrieve my car the valet manager said, "Good morning, gentlemen. Mr. Wiltgen, we sent some of your guests home in our cars last night. They were in no shape to drive. I heard it was a good party".

Maybe they would let me come back.

As I drove, it was the blind leading the partially blind. We wound around serpentine Sunset Boulevard with Chris issuing directions like, "Okay, up ahead there should be this little road on the left. There won't be a sign. It might look like a private drive. Yeah? All right turn there."

He has a sixth sense.

The morning sun burnt through the Ocean's midst. The Buddhist gardens were in bloom. Mother Nature was flaunting her expertise. The grounds were remarkable, but I was more amazed by how Chris maneuvered his way around the landscape. Somehow he knew exactly where to find statues and miniature temples erected for meditation. Chris loved the sanctuary but found its splendor in a different way than the rest of us. He found the peace and serenity quite exquisite rendering him completely at ease. It was hard to grasp his blindness.

After two hours of wandering we decided to check on the remaining party guests. Chris pointed "the way out is just ahead."

I put the car in drive and swung onto Sunset Boulevard.

A few minutes...a few miles. I don't know. Chris said something about pulling over. He sensed my low blood sugar triggering a diabetic seizure. I was out of it. My body shook so violently I could not hold the steering wheel. I didn't respond as cars sped past us in the other three lanes.

Chris reached over and put the car in park. Even though he can't see he hoped he could maneuver us to the side of the road. As cars sounded their horns, Chris realized his limitations. No matter how much he wanted to move the car to a safer location, he couldn't. Instead, he put the car in park and dragged me across two of Sunset Boulevard's four lanes. We were lucky no one ran into him or over my legs.

A stranger asked if we needed help.

Chris explained his blindness and my unconscious condition requiring several candy bars. There was no candy in my pocket. The man gave directions to a grocery store on the other side of a hedge, then drove off in our rental car.

Reese's Peanut Butter Cups. He said I fought him as he forced the candy into my mouth. It took a while before I started to come to. Suddenly, we heard a siren.

Did someone call 911?

I did not want to end up in a strange hospital. I still had guests in my hotel room. I begged Chris to hide me. He dragged me through some bushes so we could sit in a parking lot. Holding me tight he feared I might strike my head on the concrete. The noon sun tried to warm my skin, but my sugar was still so low I felt as if I were in Antarctica.

The siren got louder, then fainter, and louder again as paramedics searched Sunset for the blind guy and unconscious diabetic. When they finally gave up we found the rental car, ignition key under the floor mat, with a note wishing us well. I got in the driver's seat and drove us back to the "Pink Palace" as if nothing happened.

For all my escapades with Karen and Bobby and the opportunity to hang out with some of Hollywood's best, my dreams of moving to LA and designing homes for the rich and famous never took off.

It wasn't for the lack of trying. I put a lot of time and money into the effort.

Later in life I would receive commissions from some well-known actors, but during the interim I settled for the incredible experiences. A large part of my success in life came from the fact I was never afraid to say YES, to take chances and dream big.

I refused to let my health rule.

FOREVER IS
AS LONG AS IT LASTS

Christmas seemed to be the holiday that gave me mostly medical scenarios. On Christmas Eve Day (1997) Dr. Oyer wanted an immediate angiogram to examine my heart function. My cholesterol was within the desired range for a chronic diabetic, but his order for the test CHRISTMAS EVE meant something was wrong.

The angiogram was an outpatient procedure, but I still had to change into one of those stupid gowns.

Note to self: talk to Cynthia about designing a collection of more stylish models than the crappy blue cover-ups they give me and everyone else. That's a lot of gowns.

Wouldn't something more fashionable lift a patient's spirits? One-inch wide black and white stripes for those who identify as men. Brightly colored block print florals for people who identify as women. The interiors could be designed around them.

During pre-op, I signed an informed consent. The doctor asked if I had a Living Will or Durable Power of Attorney "in the event of death". The word "death" is used all too often in the hospital where they are supposed to make you better.. It's not very reassuring when you're the one on the gurney.

After being shaved beneath my belt line and anesthetized— the radiologist inserted a thin hollow tube into a large artery in my leg. Contrast dye revealed advanced heart disease resulting from diabetes and my control. Make that "lack of control". I was 38 years old. Two of my three arteries were so clogged they could not be opened. However, good news. The artery remaining open wrapped itself around my heart delivering oxygen-rich blood to the muscle. When the test was completed I laid flat for several hours enabling the site (where the catheter had been inserted) to clot. On discharge, the medics instructed me to avoid anything strenuous for the next 10 days. No lifting. No squatting. Nothing. No one wanted my incision to open. I could bleed to death.

There's that word again.

The next morning I schlepped my luggage through the airport and escaped to Palm Springs leaving my fucked up real world behind. I phoned Aunt Bea informing her I was on my way. We always have crazy good times together and I knew my fear and depression would quickly disappear. And it did.

But when I returned, my visits to the hospital seemed endless.

The fifth toe on my left foot became gangrenous. Fever and chills warned me something was wrong. The skin covering the toe started to break down. There were multiple wounds between the toes, smelly necrotic tissue, and exposed bone. It was like something from a horror film. I also had ulcers on the right foot. Dr. Giegerich ordered a PICC line and more antibiotics.

Why are surgeries always in the morning, I wondered en-route to another operating room. Can't they ever let me sleep in?

Researchers at Duke University concluded problems increase greatly with operations performed later in the day. Patients are more likely to develop complications from surgeries beginning after 4 pm as opposed to those starting at 8 am.

For that reason, early morning procedures are better than lying awake in a room worrying about the meaning of all this. Giegerich explained that a "digital" amputation, if necessary, would not impact my walking. Another ankle block. The doctor didn't think I needed to be put to sleep. Listening to them talk among themselves, as if I weren't there, unsettled me. I counted lightbulbs in the ceiling and prayed a bunch of "Our Fathers" and "Hail Mary's".

Just in case.

After completing a left toe incision and drainage a still-gowned Giegerich approached me. He was sorry but the toe had to come off. Debridement would not fix the osteomyelitis and advancing soft tissue infection. Not performing this amputation would only make matters worse. He was trying to save the rest of the foot.

I went home with several IV antibiotics. Like my other drugs, they too had side effects. Some were like the symptoms I experienced before they cut off the toe: fever, chills, sore throat, headache. It was difficult to know if I was improving.

What about work?

I had to go to work. After being so grossed out by what I saw every morning while changing bandages, I went to the office.

Dr. Giegerich complimented me on doing an excellent job with the wound care. Yay. And he was right. I walked the same as before even though I was missing a toe. Fortunately, it wasn't needed for balance.

One-month later Claire (we were finally on a first name basis) said my osteo was healing and I no longer needed the PICC line but within weeks I was back in his office. My right foot developed a collection of ulcers.

Not on purpose.

More osteomyelitis and septic arthritis which likely came from germs traveling through my bloodstream. Germs I probably picked up in the hospital. An increasing number of hospital infections are caused by hard to kill superbugs which developed resistance to antibiotics. My foot needed to be debrided AS SOON AS POSSIBLE.

I was having a hard time managing my diabetes because I couldn't exercise. I blamed Giegerich. He constantly reminded me to stay off my feet which resulted in higher blood sugars. Desperate to return to my office so I could worry about work instead of my feet, I hobbled back and forth to it in orthopedic oxfords I detested. I detested everything. Being a diabetic. The drugs I took for my kidney transplant. Not knowing how long my heart was going to hold out. And the fucking shoes that did not compliment my super model outfits.

Pardon my French.

Often overcome with a high fever and chills I couldn't cover myself with enough blankets to stay warm. I shook violently. My teeth chattered. I felt like shit. I would go to work every day chewing Tylenol. When I finally returned home, I was exhausted. After microwaving a bag of peas or corn for dinner, I'd fall into bed.

Battling cellulitis and osteomyelitis for years, I finally agreed to wear a "Cam Walker" on my left leg to hopefully heal the open wound. It is a big, black, chunky boot allowing patients like me, to walk by restricting movement at the ankle, thus protecting the wound. I would take it off at night using crutches to maneuver around my home and was told the boot wouldn't be needed when the problem healed.

If it healed.

My medical team repeatedly talked about amputation. Either removing half of my foot or more aggressively cutting below the knee. After a lot of self-control, an endless number of prayers and many visits with my doctors the open wound on the bottom of my foot healed. Another miracle! I was ecstatic and felt deserving of some-time away. Despite the unbearable heat (it was summer) I returned to Palm Springs. And even though I was missing parts of different toes, I was not too embarrassed to lay poolside barefoot casually draping a towel over my feet.

I was proud of the battles I survived. My scars were like a badge of courage!

One afternoon, after splashing around in the pool, I climbed out and onto my chaise lounge barely 10 feet away. Placing a towel over my head, I instantly fell asleep. I awoke to a nightmare. A pool of blood surrounded me. The 118-degree temperature made the pavement hot enough to fry an egg and burn the bottoms off both my feet.

I wrapped towels around them and hobbled to my room. I did not do a skilled job with the primitive wrapping because the carpet, from the door to the bathroom, looked like a crime scene. There was blood everywhere. With the sterile gauze and antibiotic ointment I packed, I disinfected my feet wrapping them like expensive Christmas presents

On hands and knees, I crawled around my room attempting to remove the stains from the carpet. A dozen four letter words went through my head. When finished, I climbed onto the bed and passed out.

I tried to sleep but roaring noises in my head kept me from doing so. Half-awake I thought it was background music to a bad movie playing in the room next door. The following morning, I felt awful. The racket persisted. Something was wrong. I had to get to a hospital. When I stood it was as if I'd been slung from a human sling shot. My instability was violent unlike anything I'd ever experienced. Crawling on my hands and knees again I saw remnants of blood still staining the carpet.

Outside I tried to walk but fell into a sharp prickly pear cactus. On all fours, I made my way to my rental car.

In a hospital, stripped down on a gurney with an IV, I recited my life's medical history to half a dozen nurses and doctors. After diagnosing the third degree burns on the bottom of my feet, they kept asking me to stick out my tongue as they peered into my ears. Several hours of inspection and a shot of Antivert, their opinion was vertigo.

When the drug kicked in, I felt good as new. A nurse discharged me with a prescription for the pill version and insisted I return to Chicago IMMEDIATELY and see my own physicians.

I thought vertigo was a psychological disorder; a fear of heights as in the film noir directed by Alfred Hitchcock. Who knew it could be so physical?

At home, I knew how to bandage my feet but didn't have a clue why vertigo found my head. The otolaryngologist ordered tests. His exams confirmed what I already knew. I could not hear anything with my left ear.

An electronystagmogram tested my balance. I flunked.

Blind in my left eye, now deaf in my left ear, no working kidney on that side, my left half had become my shitty side. Real shitty.

The doctor concluded the vertigo resulted from Meniere's Disease, a cause of dizziness that usually takes months or years to become evident, let alone permanent. Of course, mine was permanent in one weekend. Autoimmune illnesses have been found to produce Meniere's disease. Diabetics with peripheral neuropathy and other circulation disorders are candidates for this.

The ulcers on my feet grew out of control! Doctor Giegerich was unhappy I couldn't stay off them. With my responsibilities: clients, employees, subcontractors, etc., it was impossible. He warned the infection could contaminate my bones and was doing everything conceivable to save my foot.

I had to do my part.

IT'S A JUNGLE OUT THERE

Susan's boy toy husband was out of town in August. He went to Santorini to see his mom and dad so she needed a date for a builder association black-tie affair. She asked me, knowing I had a closet full of tuxedos and dinner jackets. It was at the Ambassador East Hotel, home of the famed Pump Room, one of my favorite playgrounds.

We rushed through the lobby happily holding hands as if we were the newlyweds, steered to the right, then up the stairs and… "SURPRISE," the crowd yelled.

I was shell-shocked.

Susan, that vixen, along with my other best friend, Bill, pulled off the greatest shocker of my life. More than 120 family members, friends, and some of my favorite clients joined me in celebrating my fortieth. People flew in from both coasts. There was a jazz band, lots of liquor, a sit-down dinner and three-tiered birthday cake decorated with a Versace Medusa emblem on top.

Years later, I learned the host and hostess were convinced the state of my current health could prevent me from celebrating future birthdays.

Jeff seemed camera shy that night. Every time the photographer gathered a group for pictures, he moved away. Could it have been his new triple processed bleach blonde hair? I kept asking him to get into a photo, but he wouldn't. And, as it turned out—it didn't matter. The photographer went to a bar afterwards, was overserved and lost the film in her struggle to get home. The digital camera age had not yet arrived.

On our way home I was on a high. Probably a sugar one. I would have to check my glucose as soon as we walked through the door. We were moving into a loft in less than two weeks. The custom work I imagined was almost done. Tumbled stone floors. Onyx doorknobs. Gold plated bathroom faucets. Egyptian temple-like door casings and pediments. Curved walls. Sheer drapery fabric with tiny little hieroglyphs printed just for me. Hieroglyphs everywhere as the backdrop for my growing collection of thousands of years-old Egyptian artifacts.

I wish my European professor, Manuel, could have seen it. Our visits with him to numerous Italian villas designed by Andrea Palladio influenced my newest home. Before this class, I visualized one long accent wall of hieroglyphs in the entry, but after seeing how Palladio's villas and palazzos were faux painted from floor-to-ceiling and wall-to-wall, I finished everything in Egyptian themed murals. In plaster, they were as authentic as a five-hundred-year-old Palladian villa in northern Italy. Suddenly I had a flashback of Frank Barbaria's home.

What would he think of it?

Jeff and I were lucky to have great friends. Still in the car I let him know we needed to put together a guest list for a Halloween costume party. I purchased two elaborately decorated Medieval princely outfits for Jeff and me while in Venice. They were like works of art. Who did he think we should invite?

Slowly he turned to me and said…

"I'm leaving."

Two major shocks in one night. And almost one car accident. You don't say stuff like that to me while I'm driving.

"I'm moving to the hair loft. I will live and work there," he continued. "I already ordered a murphy bed. I'll be gone next week."

What does one say to that?

All sorts of thoughts raced through my head. Fifteen years together. Yes, with some time-outs, but in the most recent years he never talked about anything being so bad he had to leave.

Again.

I would miss him terribly, but the reality is we are very different. He claimed I did not take care of myself. He was tired of worrying about me. Tired of the paramedics having to rush me to the hospital due to tragic episodes of low blood sugar. And I worked too much.

He didn't understand work was my distraction from the health problems that have always haunted me. Since I was 8 -years old I have thought about diabetes every day of my life.

Nonetheless, I worked hard and tried to show my friends and family a good time. I was happiest entertaining them.

I was traveling more too. And since Jeff did not want to sit on a plane for 8 or 9 hours, I took Mom along. Paris. Florence. Vincenza. Asolo. Venice. Venice. Venice.

I always wanted the best for him and tried to show him what the best could be. He had been in my life for such a long time and glimpsed parts of it no one else would ever see. He was with me when I was a nobody and witnessed my ascent in the world of design. That bond was like epoxy.

He moved from our house to his loft, and I moved into the Egyptian Temple. Which I loved. It was pure theatre. Guests who came there for the first time wondered which door Elizabeth Taylor / Cleopatra was hiding behind.

When that year ended, I was disappointed to learn I had not flown enough miles to maintain my preferred airline status which was important to me as I enjoyed the frequent upgrades to First Class. I asked Leana if she was interested in going on a far-away vacation with moi.

Yes. Despite all the changes in my life, we were still speaking to one another.

I needed approximately 7,000 miles to keep my status and told her to find a way to rack 'em up. I asked Jeff first, but once again, he said no.

Queeny (Jeff's nickname for her) worked it all out. Christmas Eve, after spending part of the holiday with my family, I went to O'Hare with my luggage and a tin filled with diet kolackies Cindy baked especially for me.

I flew to Los Angeles to meet Leana. She moved to LA after

learning things were not going to work out between us although she did like Jeff. In LA we boarded a plane to Miami where we checked into an airport hotel for a six-hour nap and five-minute shower before the next segment of our trip. This was a roundabout way to get to our destination, but the miles added up. With the time changes it was hard to decide when to take my drugs and food.

We boarded a three-hour flight to San Jose, Costa Rica but our destination was Quepos, on the Pacific Coast, which required a chartered private plane for the last leg of our trip. Leana said the quaint town was like the Mediterranean Riviera. She packed a black leather dress with gold epaulets to wear New Year's Eve which she accessorized with a feather boa. The former bird was so long it required a suitcase all its own. Thinking it would be just like sunny Acapulco in its hey-day, I bought a chartreuse Versace tuxedo with grosgrain collar and black silk shirt to ring in the New Year. And Leana booked a hilltop casita with panoramic views of the Pacific. She thought of everything.

We landed in San Jose amidst a torrential downpour. All commuter flights were canceled. How would we make it to Quepos? The weather surprised me. Where was the sun? We were approximately four-hundred miles closer to the equator than Acapulco. I did not expect such a vast climate change. We collected our bags and hailed a taxi asking the driver to take us to the private plane hangar.

There the taxi driver held his umbrella over Leana and himself as I unloaded our collection of suitcases. I made several very wet trips to get them from the cab to the metal shelter covering an assortment of planes.

"Senor Wiltgen?" I heard a voice but could not spot the person. My glasses were dripping wet and, at 2:30 pm, it was dark outside.

"Aqui arriba." The pilot waved to me from something looking like a 20-year-old crop duster, its propeller spinning.

"Hola," I did not have my Spanish phrase book handy. "At the aeropurto (I pointed) they said all flights were grounded because of the rain. Comprende?"

"Si, senor," said the pilot with a smile. And then, in his best English. "No problema para me. We go. Before it gets... no light."

I looked at Leana. Her olive-toned Macedonian complexion blanched.

"Look," I tried to sound confident. "He's the pilot. He could give-a-shit about us but he's gonna make damn sure nothing happens to him. Merry Christmas."

I loaded our bags into the plane's storage compartment. It was a crop duster. We climbed inside. There were no doors and no glass in the window openings. And no seat belts. And I'm not kidding.

The flight was 45 long minutes. San Jose is in a valley surrounded by mountain and a volcano or two. The plane climbed straight up. I grabbed the metal framing. Leana held me so tightly her press-on fingernails cut through my shirt and the skin on my back. We were encased in nimbostratus clouds. I tried to get my bearings. Suddenly, a mountain loomed straight ahead. Couldn't be seen a second earlier. As the pilot turned 90-degrees I was looking down 7,500 feet at a riverbed and many jagged edges. Leana was on top of me, but I couldn't grab her. I was too busy holding on for my own dear life.

"I think I'm gonna be sick," she said.

"Just hang your head out the window or door," I tried joking though it was no laughing matter. It *was* a long way down and I didn't see any parachutes.

Finally, the downpour began to diminish. The sun started peeking through the dense blanket of dark gray clouds. We began our decent. The blue Pacific was in the distance. The ground below was a beautiful shade of green. A jungle. Which is exactly where our pilot landed. In the middle of nowhere. Literally nowhere and it was still drizzling.

He helped retrieve the bags placing them under a giant elephant ear tree to protect them from the rain and mud. I turned to Leana.

"Now what?" I asked. This was nothing like Acapulco.

"They should be here shortly..." she did not sound too convincing and our only contact with civilization just took off.

"Who are they?" I kindly demanded.

"THEY. The people from the hotel. I told them we would land around 4:00. It is 3:40 now." She looked at her rubber Swatch watch.

"Okay. We are in the middle of a jungle. No phone. No phone booth. No hut with a door and glass in the windows to protect us from the jaguars, panthers and 22 varieties of poisonous snakes slithering around. I'm just saying."

I started to pace in a useless pair of espadrilles. Where were my combat boots?

"Do you want bug spray?" Leana worried I would be bitten by a mosquito and my suppressed immune system would not be able to fight malaria or dengue. Jaguars kill fewer people than pesky little mosquitos. I closed my eyes and held my nose as she sprayed me with Deep Woods Off containing 25 percent DEET.

It seemed like forever before the rusted, mud covered, Jeep hacked its way through the foliage. The Huetares Indian driver asked in thickly accented Spanish if we were Senor y Senora Wiltgen. We nodded anxiously. We would have done so even if he said he was going to tie us to a post and burn us alive. He picked up our bags, apologizing for being late.

"Puente out debido a toda la lluvia," he tried to explain. We strained to understand. Something about a bridge and all the rain.

"Si, of course," we nodded. I wanted food, maybe some of Cindy's diet kolacky's, a hot shower and bed.

Slowly we plowed through the jungle while troops of white-faced capuchin monkeys, best known as organ grinders' companions, followed swinging from overhead tree branches. A three-toed sloth hanging upside down stared at us. Brightly colored birds also studied the Americanos del Norte traveling through their jungle.

Despite the potential threat of some snake falling out of the branches overhead, I was in awe of the raw beauty we observed between the raindrops dancing on the trailing leaves. It was not like Acapulco. It never rained when I was there. The mountains kept the rain away. It was humid, as in "very", but always sunny.

By the time we reached the hotel the rain was much heavier than when we landed. I almost missed the office. It and the rooms were archaic little huts enveloped in dense hillside vegetation. Uwa, our driver, helped carry our luggage into the oficina. The girl behind the desk greeted us with a big smile. Our room was at the top of the hill she explained tilting her head high. She gazed out the window pointing to an endless flight of broken concrete stairs.

"Donde esta el portero?" I inquired.

"Oh, no senor," she frowned. "Lo siento."

Tired beyond belief, I begrudgingly seized some of our bags. Leana grabbed her handbag and the box containing her boa and together we schlepped our possessions to the hilltop casita—the one with the views of the Pacific. The stairs were transformed into a gentle but treacherous waterfall with all sorts of creepy crawly critters mixed with the agua. Without an umbrella we climbed the stairway to heaven.

More than 200 effen slippery steps.

Much to our surprise or NOT the door to our room was unlocked. That explained why there wasn't a telephone or TV. So much for calling home. I dropped the bags on the Saltillo tile floor and slid down the hill for the few remaining pieces. When I returned soaking wet, I shed my clothes.

Leana said it wasn't *that* bad meaning it was terrible.

The glassless windows had 4-inch-thick wood blinds adjustable for privacy. The rafters supporting the pitched roof sat on the exterior walls, but there was nothing between them to seal the interior. At least the bathroom had a door, but with louvers that were separating from the frame.

I started to unpack and organize syringes, insulin and other drugs, but first a kolacky. Maybe two or three. Even Cindy's diet ones are addicting. I dug through the suitcase for the round Christmas tin in which she so thoughtfully packaged them. When I opened it, **shock of life,** the tin was packed with *dinner rolls.* Not the sugar free jelly filled cookies I saw 30 hours ago. Ray. One of his practical jokes. I'd get him when I returned.

Leana screamed.

I ran to the bathroom. Standing away from the sink she tried to point though her fists were clenched. A spotted lime green frog with bulging silvery-white eyes poked his head up through the drain. WTF. The wastepipe must have fed directly into the jungle. Good to know. We'd keep the drain tightly closed when not in use. I turned on the hot water, rinsed Kermit away and stood guard as Leana washed her face. Then it was my turn. She went back to the bedroom.

Two minutes later she screeched even louder as she tried to open the door to escape.

"WHAT?" I questioned madly. I was tired and...OH MY GOD. Leana folded back the blankets on the bed only to uncover a huge, hairy Tarantula as big as my hand when my fingers were fully extended. I grabbed a book and smashed the creature all over the recently laundered sheet.

Welcome to Costa Rica.

I wore combat boots to bed every night with a pair of jeans, gym socks rolled over the hem, and a long-sleeved sweatshirt. I was not leaving myself exposed. Too bad I didn't pack a turtleneck or scarf.

Before deciding it was safe for us to go to sleep Leana went outside and lit mosquito coils around the perimeter of our shanty—one every four or five feet. She brought boxes of them which was a good move because we needed them.

We quickly learned breakfasts were an exercise in protecting our food from the wildlife. Those pesky little monkeys sat on the fence nearby and, when we weren't looking, jumped to our table and confiscated a banana or piece of toast. They really liked it with butter and jelly! If we dropped something on the floor while fighting off the monkeys, a three-foot iguana would dart out of the foliage to collect the remains. Our waiter stood guard. When he saw the reptiles, he'd grab them by their tails and hurl them back into the dense foilage.

After breakfast I'd go to the beach. Leana would venture across the river into Manuel Antonio National Park to sunbathe au natural. On a log. In the jungle. All alone. A naked woman. Repeatedly, I asked her not to go. It was dangerous, but she said she could take care of herself although I heard she had some help.

In her skimpy "dental floss" like bathing suit, Leana met many people from the greater Los Angeles area on our beach. "Don't you and your husband just love it here?" someone asked as we waded in the Pacific.

"Are you kidding me?" I answered. Perhaps too quickly. "My idea of ruffing it is in a casita at Las Brisas (Acapulco). Each casita has its own swimming pool cantilevered one above the other. Drivers in pink jeeps appear out of nowhere to transport you around the property, to the beach club or downtown.

We were definitely overdressed on New Year's Eve. To compliment Leana's feather boa I purchased a Versace tuxedo just for the trip. However, Quepos was NOT the Riviera of the Pacific. Everyone else was dressed in jeans and t-shirts. But, we looked good. No. We looked great.

January 1 may have been the beginning of the New Year, but January 2 was time to truly celebrate. We were leaving. Our plane with familiar pilot landed in the same middle of nowhere for our return to San Jose. Queeny decided to stay in Costa Rica. See what kind of trouble she could find. I was taking the short route to Chicago via Miami.

Landing on the tarmac at Miami International Airport, I got down on my hands and knees to kiss the runway.

WE ARE FAMILY

At one time or another almost everyone in my family worked at John Robert Wiltgen Design, Inc. It truly was a family business. People liked that—those people being us.

Regina started her career with me when she was 6-years old. At that time, I had an office on the 17th floor of the Merchandise Mart. I'd send her to the bank on the first floor to make deposits. Then she'd buy each of us a frozen yogurt cone from Mrs. O'Leary's Yogurt Shop. Sometimes she would return fabric samples to showrooms on another floor in the massive two-block long building. She was a big help and not afraid. I wasn't afraid for her either OR was I just plain stupid?

All three of my sister Cindy's daughters worked for me at different times as they were growing up. Savannah was a full-time employee for 18-months and learned more from her co-workers than her uncle. Her younger sisters worked summers and holidays.

Mom's sister, my aunt Mary Lou, worked with us for almost six years. Her husband, also Jeff, left her unceremoniously after 25 years of marriage—the same summer my Jeff left me. The *Summer of Jeff's* we called it somewhere over the Atlantic on our way to Italy.

My professor loved her. Our class of 30 students traveled throughout northern Italy for half a month and every night he sat at our dinner table. We were heartbroken to learn he died of a brain aneurism several months later.

Mom, I mean Jean, and I loved having Mary Lou working with us. She went to the Mart to select the most unusual fabric and wallpaper samples for me to consider for our clients. She has two great eyes. Oftentimes she accompanied me on potential client interviews. She is picturesque and men love looking at her.

Once we met with a developer about an opportunity to design the lobby, common areas, and models of a new development.

I wanted to make a good impression and decided a stylish pair of loafers were in order. By coincidence I just purchased a pair at Versace in Beverly Hills. They were an innovative black leather dress shoe with a flap velcroed across the top, no laces. I had to have them.

Mary Lou and I looked chic and stunning riding in the back of a yellow cab. Before the meeting we needed to stop at the Mart. My aunt and I talked all the way there, so my attention was on our conversation. I paid the fare, closed the door behind us, and hurriedly stepped out onto the sidewalk. Something wasn't right. I looked down and couldn't believe what my one good eye saw.

Or didn't see.

One of my brand-new shoes was missing. I asked Mary Lou if that's what she saw, hoping I was hallucinating. She stared. The innovative shoe must have slipped off in the back seat of the cab without my feeling anything. And the cab was gone.

I have chronic neuropathy and therefore no feeling in my feet. Doctors are always sticking needles in them, asking "Do you feel this? No? What about this?" as the needle inches up my leg. Once, I watched Dianne Sawyer walk on hot coals on *Good Morning America* and thought maybe she has neuropathy too.

What were Mary Lou and I to do? Should she walk in as eye-candy, so no one noticed me hobbling with one shoe? No. We taxied back to my loft to fetch a less showy pair of shoes for the interview, even though it meant arriving late.

When we entered the meeting, at the conference table sat the developer and all his minions in suits, ties, and their best shoes. Good thing I wore an eye-catching, business-looking, suit and tie. I told everyone the truth which produced questionable smiles. They never heard *that* story before.

Whether our proposal was not what they were looking for, or my emergency shoes were a letdown after the dazzle of my suit, we'll never know. When we learned a few days later we didn't get the job Mary Lou and I laughed so hard we cried and that made it all worthwhile.

My brother Ray worked with me from the time I shined shoes in taverns. An entrepreneur himself, he was a big part of John Robert Wiltgen Design, Inc. Having an MBA, his professional advice came in handy. When I received the commission to design a project in Africa, he traveled across the Atlantic with me and helped create documents needed by my client and his team of advisors.

Mom worked in the design biz too for 17 years. During our lunches we talked about work and a more important subject. Family.

SOMETHING ABOUT JANE SEYMOUR

My publicists often scheduled interviews for me with design magazine editors in New York City. I frequently stayed at the then new, chic and stunning Hudson Hotel in Midtown Manhattan.

By coincidence, "Miss Hollywood" once stayed there at the same time. She was directing an art exhibit for actress, Jane Seymour at a mall in Hackensack, NJ. We checked in together even though we came from separate cities. But we weren't the only ones dazzled by the wonders of the Hudson. Our friend, Jennifer Nicholson, was at the far end of the 50-foot registration counter. I poked Karen then yelled "Hey Jennifer..."

"Wow. What are you two doing here?" she asked sounding like a valley girl even though she lived in Brentwood.

Looking as if we rendezvoused for a steamy out-of-town tryst, Karen improvised, "Jenn, you caught us. I'm so embarrassed. John and I are lovers. He should have kept his mouth shut," she grabbed my arm, "and you wouldn't have noticed us. Please, I'm begging you...don't tell Bobby."

Karen was good. Even I believed her. Had she not loved art so much I would have urged her to go in front of the camera like her husband. Jenn gave us a bewildered look as we accepted our keys.

The moment our elevator door closed we broke into laughter. Who was the first-person Jenn would tell? Bobby, of course. Karen phoned her husband asking him to play along.

Who'd have thought we'd encounter her 2,500 miles from home? The universe was toying with us.

Karen left for Hackensack early the next morning to supervise the installation of Jane's artwork. She slid a note under my door wishing me well with my interview and invited me to New Jersey to meet Jane.

My interview was a total waste of the time and the money it cost to travel to New York. At the top of our discussion, the officious editor asked if I read her publication. She said her magazine was marketed to "white trash."

Honest.

I tried to hide my disbelief. It may have been true. And I never catered to that market. I just went where my publicist sent me. But Ms. Editor-in-Chief could have been more tactful in defining her subscribers. Knowing the answer, she closed our meeting by asking what homes I designed for do-it-yourselfers fitting that category. I thanked her for her time and walked out. Fuming.

For 20 years, not counting the Frank Barbaria finishing school or the Byron, Wiltgen and Associates junior college, I worked diligently to develop and maintain my luxury brand. Since the beginning I provided excellent service, entertained my clients at dinner and black-tie affairs, participated in their non-for-profit endeavors, sent custom greeting cards for every Hallmark holiday, and purchased gifts to show my appreciation hoping these efforts (in addition to my creative design concepts) would make them ecstatic. My customers expected the very best and they knew I lived to create magnificence for them.

Leaving the editor's Broadway office, my face was beet red. I wasn't mad at the editor; I was livid with my publicist. She should have qualified this magazine before wasting days of my time. I phoned Sharon, the publicist, to share the CliffsNotes of the disastrous meeting. She laughed. Over the phone I heard fresh ice cubes refilling her glass. Furious, I hung up.

I decided to go to Hackensack where I found the British-born actress warm and friendly. I was taken by her assertive use of color and the interpretative views from her manor house in the UK. I bought two of Jane's watercolors. They were lovely.

Karen introduced us. "Jane. Meet John Robert Wiltgen. John, Jane Seymour. John is a world-famous interior designer who's won all sorts of awards and has an amazing art collection including an original Henry Moore drawing once owned by Helena Rubenstein. He just purchased two of your watercolors."

Jane, born Joyce Penelope Wilhemena Frankenberg, seemed genuinely pleased with my selections. She chose elements from each as patterns for two scarves, part of the Jane Seymour Signature Collection of women's fashions being presented to the press the following day. She invited me to attend.

Karen styled and shot several photographs of Jane with me. Then Jane moved on to schmooze (her father was a Jewish obstetrician) with other customers.

Miss Hollywood kept working, promising to phone me with the details.

The next morning, the details meant meeting Karen and Jane in a ballroom at the Palace Hotel. When Karen saw me in the crowd of mostly press, she pulled me toward the front of the room. Unexpectedly, Jane told the group a famous, internationally acclaimed designer, purchased two original works of her art which inspired some scarves.

She pointed to me.

Flying home, I thought about hosting a Chicago exhibit of Jane's art. While in a cab, I phoned my publicist despite still being mad at her.

"Well, I think it is a fabulous idea. Would she do it?" more ice cubes tumbled around her glass. It wasn't even noon in Chicago.

"I have no idea, but as soon as Karen's plane lands I will call her."

My mind raced 100 miles per hour. Working fast it could be a Christmas gala. We would schedule interviews with the press. Print and TV. It had to happen no later than the first week of December. After that everyone is busy with office and family events.

Miss Hollywood loved the idea. Jane agreed. Her holiday schedule was tight, but she could stop in Chicago on her way home from an engagement in Toronto.

Deal.

During the next three days, I inspected hotel suites befitting King Henry VIII's wife, Jane Seymour. I met the general managers of Chicago's five-star hotels. They all wanted Jane as their guest, but the holiday season rooms suitable for a Bond girl *(Live and Let Die)* were already booked.

The Drake offered the perfect space, and it was available. Not only that. The Princess Diana Suite, nearly 5,000-square-feet, provides its guests with romantic views of the Oak Street Beach.

Now, where would we display Jane's art?

A duplex owned by a client was empty while they awaited my summary of the costs to combine their duplex with the adjoining one. They were thrilled at the prospect of hosting a party for the well-known celebrity.

Health-wise. I had another PICC line to go along with another foot infection. Every day I wore ugly orthopedic oxfords. Not at all stylish, but for the Seymour party, I squeezed my bandaged feet into a pair of Versace loafers for an excruciatingly long seven hours.

Jane knows firsthand the effects of diabetes and has been active in public campaigns to help patients come to terms with their illness. Her grandmother was a type 2 diabetic who succumbed to the effects of the disease losing her eyesight and developing gangrene in a leg later removed.

December 1, 2001 was the date Jane confirmed for the exhibit. It was by invitation only. More than 300 acceptances swept in.

Jane was stunned to see so much of her work on exhibit in the gallery we created. It overflowed with clients, family, friends and the press. Every local newspaper and magazine editor was anxious to attend. We even scheduled a TV interview the following morning.

Jane was extremely gracious and autographed cassettes and VHS tape boxes brought by many. She posed in photographs with almost everyone. That's a lot of smiles.

The children at the local Ronald McDonald House smiled a lot too. They received two vans loaded with toys we asked guests to bring to the party, gift wrapped, as admission.

Her right hand ached by the end of the evening. She elegantly worked it signing so many dedications. And despite my spreading infection, I was on top of the world.

WHO COULD ASK FOR ANYTHING MORE?

My war with osteomyelitis seemed like the Thirty Years' War fought in Europe between 1618 to 1648 leaving more than 800,000 soldiers and civilians dead.

Despite the high powered IV antibiotics, the sores on my left foot continued to grow. The one on my right foot was smaller but deeper. Each time I saw the doctor, he told me to keep my weight off my feet.

What was I to do? Walk on my hands?

Surgeries became routine. Once, with his back to me, Giegerich used a power saw to remove more of yours truly. When the bleeding stopped, I returned to my office.

Night and day, I continually ran a low-grade fever. If I took enough acetaminophen it helped me make it through work and I thought I felt okay; not that I really knew how okay felt anymore.

Dangerous bacteria were present when the doctor mentioned a forefoot amputation. Again. The idea made me sick. I couldn't imagine my foot without any toes even though some were already missing.

To avoid thinking about it, I decided to go to Europe. The doctor grimaced as he explained I would remain on IV antibiotics. If serious chills or fever developed, I'd need to go to a hospital there OR arrange for urgent travel home.

I bought travel insurance.

My close friends Bill, and his fiancé Leslie, finally chose July 3, 2002, to be married. (I say "finally" because she patiently waited for Bill's divorce from Georgia to be concluded.) Their destination wedding was in Arezzo; the setting for the movie *Life Is Beautiful.*

That was the only reason I was going to Europe.

Susan (Tjarksen) and I were the matron of honor and best man. Schlepping a carry-on bag filled with IV antibiotics packed in dry ice, sterile gauze, medical tape, PICC line supplies, and other pharmaceuticals, I was committed to being there for my friends. They were always there for me.

Susan, her 4-year-old daughter, Ellie, and I flew together. Somewhere over the Atlantic the vivacious preschooler provided in-flight entertainment, standing at the front of the cabin singing the Greek national anthem to her first-class audience. Her father is from Santorini, so Ellie traveled back and forth to Greece from the time she was 16-months. Maybe I encouraged her but as we left the plane multiple passengers said it was great my daughter was bi-lingual at such a young age. I agreed.

It is so much easier to be a part-time father to someone else's kid.

Checking into our hotel, the bride's and groom's family members were getting well-acquainted in a magnificent 15th century villa Bill reserved for the occasion. The three of us joined the group for dinner the next evening, then hopped a train to Venice early the following morning. Susan had never been there, and I adored giving her a private tour of one of my favorite cities. Ellie enjoyed the sites as much as did we. Piazza San Marco, Saint Mark's Basilica, the Doge's Palace, but particularly the gondola rides.

She called me Johnny Versace, producing numerous confused stares. The late fashion mogul was murdered five years earlier on the steps of his Miami palazzo. Staff members were crazed when we went into the Venetian Versace as the principessa continually referred to me by the bastardized version of their iconic founder's name. But that didn't prevent them from selling me a suit and pair of shoes which I wore to dinner that evening with my girls.

Dinner on the rooftop of the Danieli Excelsior Palace provides one of Venice's most celebrated views of the Canale Grande lined with Renaissance and Gothic palazzos tucked between massive limestone cathedrals. Both Susan and I were extremely sentimental over our good fortune of being able to share this exceptional time together. We wished it would never end but I had to get back to my hotel room for another round of IV antibiotics.

We were late returning to Arezzo for the wedding. The train did not move fast enough to meet our timetable. Before dressing, I had to shower and another hour of drugs to absorb. The bride and groom could not be married without us, even with the

Mayor presiding. It was an amazing wedding reminiscent of a classic, black and white movie, maybe starring a young Bette Davis and Humphrey Bogart. Despite what the doctor told me I was so happy I went. The only regretful moment was…NO. Not our being late. During the cocktail hour the orchestra played *Georgia on my Mind*. I emphatically ordered them to STOP. Georgia, Bill's former wife, was NOT on his mind!

Upon my return, I checked in with Dr. Giegerich. Despite all my walking around Venice, Arezzo and assorted airports, he said my foot looked better. Only God knew why the wound was smaller with less swelling and redness. But then, the x-ray showed a fracture of the mid and forefoot and new bone formation.

Charcot foot.

An echocardiogram confirmed my heart was not involved in the recurrent infections. No excess fluid appeared in the sac surrounding it. Additional liquid from osteomyelitis can put pressure on the heart leading to heart failure or death. Many diabetic complications can lead to death.

Try putting that out of your mind.

As I was changing bandages one morning, a piece of bone fell out of my foot. It freaked me out. I never saw anything like that happen in a scary movie, not even the ever-popular zombie films.

What was happening to me?

I was literally falling apart. Were my bones going to continue leaving me until there was nothing left but a pound of flesh? I didn't want to live my life in fear, but sometimes I couldn't help it.

The next few years brought little change. To celebrate the *pulling of one of the PICC Lines* a friend and I escaped to Nice. My blind friend, Chris, introduced Jimmy to me and we became besties. He was in the store fixture business with some national department stores as clients. Jimmy also dabbled in real estate. We shared a lot of the same interests, and he was an awesome travel partner. Spontaneous.

On this trip we stayed at a resort in the French countryside. I was thrilled to be surrounded by rolling hills, each topped by its own little hamlet, where we did nothing.

Especially not visiting doctors.

After a week of that, we went to St. Tropez to do something. I drove. We stayed in a 19th century haunted chateau on a hilltop with spectacular views of the Mediterranean and surrounding vineyards. Since I had never been, we explored a nude beach. *That* view didn't thrill me. And I didn't take my shoes off.

My left foot was treated to more out-patient surgeries. I should have let them cut the whole thing off, but my vanity won over while, ever so slowly, my foot disappeared piece by piece.

***

In February 2004 I was rushed by ambulance to Northwestern Memorial Hospital. When anyone's glucose is way above normal, the blood thickens which can result in a heart attack. Just ask me, although I don't remember much. While reloading my insulin pump, I neglected to remove the protective cover from the long, thin insertion needle. Therefore, no insulin was delivered to my body causing my glucose level to rise as I slept.

I don't remember how I got to the hospital. Jeff said I was in a stupor when I phoned him for help. He dialed 911. Surgeons inserted two stents to keep open my one artery. Before the operation, my nephrologist had me hydrated to protect my kidney. I gained more than 40 pounds of water weight and ballooned to a size which kept me from seeing my johnson. Mom was afraid I would die and started calling family and friends.

As bad as they seemed at the time, and even now when I reflect on these circumstances, my personal problems did not slow things down at my office. I had twenty-nine projects in different phases of development and installation all at once.

Despite long, flowing lists of hospital and doctor visits over the past few years, I acquired eleven design awards for recently completed projects including a Silver Design Award for a built-in, home office/library. A Gold Design Award for a contemporary loft living room. A Gold Key Award for Outstanding Design of a model home. First Place in an international design competition for the master bathroom in the house in Rancho Santa Fe, CA. The combination of them certainly elevated my reputation. I was forty-three, still alive and loving my work.

THE GERMAN POPE, THE WEDDING AND THE NOSE JOB

Twenty years later I was still trying to repay Mom for the second life she gave me unconditionally.

What else could I do for her?

Then, while reading the Dan Brown book *Angels and Demons,* it came to me. Rome. I would take her to see the Pope. The German one.

It was not as easy as buying tickets for the Academy Awards from a bookie. I really had to work on this. I lucked out when I discovered one of my Italian born vendors was uber Catholic and had connections at the Vatican. He contacted a well-placed compadre, and eventually we had a date to see the Pontiff.

Mom cried more than any other time in her life. She was so happy. As we waited with hundreds to see Pope Benedict XVI, I passed out from low blood sugar.

Right there in Vatican City.

Thank goodness Jimmy was with us. He tried forcing candy down my throat but being obstinate, especially when my sugar is 15 or 20, that didn't work. When he realized he needed God's help he ran to find the Swiss Guard leaving me with Mom and her new husband Marty.

Mom got married to the kindest guy. This man loves and adores Mom. He put her on a pedestal so high she would break an arm if she fell off it.

Regaining consciousness, I gazed up at the clouds asking if I was in heaven. The angel replied, "pretty damn close my son." When he told me I was in the Vatican infirmary I sat up. The trompe-l'oeil clouds painted on the vaulted ceiling seemed so realistic they certainly fooled my eye. Without delay I was returned to an anxious Mom, Marty and Jimmy in an electric car resembling the Popemobile.

"C'est un miracle," cried a handful of French worshippers who had been praying for me on their knees.

"It wasn't a miracle. It was sugar water," I replied. Mom gave me a hard tap. Once she knew I was okay she ordered me to be quiet.

***

In July I scooped up my four nieces and whisked them off to LA to work on our tans prior to Regina's wedding a few days later. Their parents were scared to death.

What did I know about parenting four young girls, ages 8 through 16? What if my blood sugar took a dive and I passed out? OR, even worse, what if I developed a fever and needed to be hospitalized?

My family is great. They have seen me through countless problems. That is the problem. They are too aware.

Ray's wife, Gail, suggested she fly to LA with us and stay in a different hotel (if I insisted). That way there would be someone close by to save the day if it needed saving. I said no. I promised the moms and dads nothing would happen. And in the unlikely chance something went wrong with me one of the kids could call Jimmy or Regina or Miss Hollywood. After some persuasive lobbying the parents agreed.

Tony, my driver, met us at the bottom of the escalator at LAX. I did not want to pass out while driving a rental car with my four young passengers.

We had connecting rooms at the Beverly Hills Hotel where I knew excellent care would be given the girls if someone had to call 911 for me. Immediately after check-in I taught Gabriella how to order room service. Picking up the phone, telling a stranger what she wanted to eat and having it show up 20 minutes later fascinated the 8-year-old.

We spent our days poolside where the girls ordered "virgin" Pina coladas and margaritas all day. Our cabana was between those occupied by Keanu Reeves and, on the other side, Donald and Melania Trump and their new son, Baron. The Donald wore a different polyester leisure suit poolside each day.

Cassandra complained one day her stomach ached. Could it be too many sweet drinks, French fries, hamburgers and all the other crap I let her eat? How did I know kids get sick from eating too much junk food? It seemed to me they did that all the time.

Or was that me?

We were elegantly bronzed for the wedding in California's picturesque Edna Valley. The wildflowers of San Louis Obispo were in full bloom painting a beautiful backdrop for the ceremony. The sun shone brightly on the bride and groom. Maybe it was a little hot during the ceremony but as soon as the sun set behind the mountains, it cooled off. I walked the bride down the aisle. Ray read a scripture passage. After dinner, I sang a few songs with the band. Mom cried, a lot. And I did not pass out once that whole week.

***

When I pass out from low blood sugar, I do a damn good job. My best performance took place several months after the wedding. Unconscious, I somehow crawled from the bedroom to my bathroom of the Egyptian Temple. I don't know why I went that way when the food was in the other direction. In the bathroom, having violent spasms, I hit my face on the stone floor breaking my nose. The pool of blood I discovered after finally coming to is how I know that. Bleeding all over the bedroom carpet, I somehow made my way to the kitchen and stuffed myself with everything in the fridge.

Still in the wee hours of the morning, Chris, my visiting home nurse (not my blind friend Chris) arrived to change the PICC line dressing. When I opened the door, she nearly fainted. She said I was going to the Emergency Room as soon as she finished, which was exactly what I did not want.

"Either you go to the hospital OR I'm calling your mother." She knew where to stick the knife. Not wanting Mom to worry

I conceded, but first I made Chris take my picture to share with friends.

The doorman of my condominium building must have been exceedingly worried as he helped me into a cab. He called Mom to tell her something happened. I was covered in blood and on my way to the emergency room.

The next day, I went to see a plastic surgeon wanting him to do something to my nose so it wouldn't need to be broken again later. The doctor removed the bandages taped to my face. My nose was swollen and tender. Both eyes were black. He said I did a good job of giving myself a nasal fracture. Without warning, he put his thumbs on both sides of the broken nose, aligning the cartilage.

OH MY GOD! That hurt.

He said I should not have difficulty breathing and, in his humble opinion, would not need plastic surgery to improve its appearance. I would heal. I was going to be fine. And maybe a little more butch!

TAKE A LOAD
OFF YOUR FEET

Five and a half years after burning the soles of my feet, my left foot was still a mess. No longer expecting improvement I became accustomed to daily showers with a plastic bag wrapped and taped around my leg to prevent water, perhaps contaminated, from further infecting the wound. Perplexed, Dr. Giegerich suggested I try Hyperbaric Oxygen Treatments (HBOT).

HBOT provides the patient to pure oxygen in a sealed chamber. Wounds need oxygen to heal. The hemophiliac son of favorite clients experienced success in healing a stubborn sore with the help of hyperbaric oxygen treatments. Their endorsement gave me the confidence to proceed.

The cost of 20 treatments was $90,000.00. That freaked me out because, prior to Obama care, my insurance policy had a cap on health care expenses, and I was running low on available payment dollars. Except for chopping off my leg, I had few choices and I was still attached to it.

I worried about the treatment since it can cause hearing loss. Already deaf in one ear, I was terrified about losing it in the other. I didn't want to become the male version of Helen Keller.

Being sick so much of the time made my underlying depression affect every waking minute of every day. I tried so hard not to let it show. In the darkest caverns of my brain, I kept thinking 100 units of insulin would polish me off nicely. But I couldn't do that to Mom. And I believed my clients and staff needed me.

That is what kept me going.

Several preliminary visits to the Clinic were needed before treatment began. They provided a wound vac to stimulate tissue growth. In a backpack with its hose visibly climbing up my pants it traveled everywhere with me. The constant irritating whirring noise drove me crazy.

It also drained me of nutrients, so I needed supplements, some of which interacted with my prescription drugs. The doctor warned I would feel more tired than usual.

After the first week, the wound VAC had not performed any miracles. The doctor asked if I turned it off. That thought did enter my mind, but I left it on hoping for positive results. The second week, the ulcer was debrided with expectations it would heal "faster".

My first HBOT was Monday, January 29, 2007. A nurse explained its potential complications. Fatigue, lightheadedness, rupture of the middle ear, sinus damage, vision changes, and oxygen poisoning which can cause lung failure, fluid in the lungs, or seizures.

I undressed, removed the vacuum pump, bandages and changed into—yes one of those gowns I hate. The technician helped me onto a gurney which slid into a clear plexiglass coffin-like chamber. It was locked and sealed leaving no visible means of escape unless you were Houdini.

He told me to relax.

I was sealed inside a clear coffin like Eva Peron and he wanted me to relax?

The suspended TV hung over my feet. Someone suggested I bring a movie, so on day one I brought *She's So Lovely.*

I talked to the technician as oxygen filled the tank. Slowly the pressure increased to 2.5 times above normal. My ears popped.

"Are you okay" the tech asked through an intercom.

"If I was okay, I wouldn't be here."

The treatment lasted approximately two hours including depressurizing the chamber. I did not watch one minute of the movie, instead I fell asleep. The tech saw the whole thing and said it was great. An exam was required when the treatment ended. Another doctor checked my blood pressure, heart rate, ear drums, and wound. I was cautioned against putting weight on the foot and left on crutches.

Two weeks after starting HBOT, Russell and Taylor Armstrong invited me to the Grammys. I invested money in a promising start up company Russell represented. That is how we met. Though fighting a high fever, I couldn't miss a possible opportunity to finally design a home in Beverly Hills. I asked my friend, Bill, if I could borrow his wife, Leslie, as my date.

I arranged this trip last minute, so Tony, my driver, was busy chauffeuring someone else. Instead, I was lucky to find a limo driver who I booked for 24-hours in LaLa Land. Henry met us at the airport wearing khaki pants and a short-sleeved Izod pullover. His 10-year-old bottle green Lincoln Town Car stood out like a blistered thumb. All we could do was laugh.

We changed into formal attire at Jimmy's West Hollywood penthouse condominium. Wearing a remarkable black and white-striped bodice with a floral print skirt and train, Leslie turned heads. We met Russell, Taylor, and their friends at Chateau Marmont, a fairytale-like castle on a hill.

Between awards and performances Taylor and I talked about home design. She and her venture capitalist husband were shopping for a house. Leslie told Taylor about the three homes I designed for them. One was more striking than the other. Taylor asked if I would work with her and Russell once they found a house.

Back home, I resumed my hyperbaric oxygen treatments. In early March, the supervising doctor was pleased with the progress prescribing 10 more treatments. I had 17 HBOTs to date. The wound looked good. He called it "pretty".

How can a wound be "pretty"?

However, the CAM walker, wound VAC, and HBOTs did nothing except rob me of the quality life I wanted. Sick of it all. And sick of my daily two hours in the coffin I couldn't take it anymore. I turned into a madman as I ripped the doctor a new one.

When Russell Armstrong phoned, I returned to my old, sweet self. They found a house he believed, with my help, could become their showplace. It was a Georgian on Sunset Boulevard two or three blocks west of the Beverly Hills Hotel. The inside needed work. So did the grounds. It was a stellar location. Wanting to reconfirm my interest we scheduled a date for me to inspect it.

The doctors bequeathed the same instructions they provided for years. Stay off my left leg. Change the bandages daily. Don't get the dressing wet. Elevate it as much as possible. But I had a plane to catch and a house to examine.

The Armstrongs and I liked the house they found and for a while it was my latest distraction. We developed plans in phases increasing the 6,000-square-foot home to 10,000-square-feet. Phase 1 included a master suite above the four-car garage. In Phase 2 the garage would be converted into an ultra-sophisticated, state-of-the-art theater, remodel the kitchen and make other changes to the ground floor. Once we completed that phase, a new detached four-car garage with a guest suite above would be built to reflect the architecture of the main house. Finally, the landscaping could be attacked. It was an awesome long-term opportunity for JRWD. One that would be very visible.

During one site visit I discovered the nanny sanding the hardwood floors. Russell said she was a multi-tasker and would do an amazing job.

"The floors shouldn't be done until the construction of the new master suite is finished. I haven't applied for a permit. We are 9 to 12 months from scheduling the restoration of the floors." That was my professional opinion. I never heard of a nanny multitasking like this.

Change the diapers and get back to the hardwood!

"John, we wanted a few things done so we could entertain *before* the work begins. That's why she is doing this now," Russell replied. Then he went to his Mont Blanc Meisterstuck black leather brief case and pulled out a jewelry box. "I have to show you this..." He was trying to distract me with a striking pair of diamond earrings and matching necklace. They were invited to a party at Buckingham Palace, he said, and Taylor needed something "special" to wear.

Meanwhile, the hole in the bottom of my foot was bigger than ever. Dull, brownish, and dry to the touch the exposed bone did not look healthy. One of my doctors suggested surgical "intervention", his less frightening term for amputation. That procedure, no matter what anyone called it, kept creeping up. To me it was still unacceptable. I was advised to visit my other doctors for their opinions.

My infectious disease doctor, who I love, agreed. She knew I still had a crush on my deformed, monstrous looking foot and frowned as she too recommended a below the knee amputation. But, I should discuss my options with all my doctors.

Each doctor deferred me to someone else. Were they afraid of me? Reluctantly, I returned to Dr. Giegerich praying his opinion would be somewhat uplifting. We discussed the other doctors' concerns and recommendations. Giegerich did not believe any part of the foot was salvageable. He agreed with them.

Fuck!

It would take four or five months to recover BEFORE I could be fitted for a prosthesis, several months to fabricate one, and then, I'd need physical therapy.

How would my business survive? HOW WOULD I SURVIVE? So many parts of me were good for nothing. I just wanted to work, have fun and entertain my clients and friends.

I was unwilling to proceed with having half my leg chopped off. I couldn't imagine not having two legs—even though the one was so gross looking. At that point death seemed a better option than having one cut off. I didn't want to wear a prosthesis. Gravely, Claire said the situation became life threatening.

I would take my chances. That was my response. I had done so my entire life.

I needed to escape to my unreal world. I thought I'd go to LA for a week or so and then Europe. But even though I dreamed about it, I didn't go anywhere. The severity of the situation made me too afraid.

What if things worsened?

I booked fewer appointments at work, stayed off my feet as much as possible, even stood on my head! And I took it easy, hoping and *praying* to save my leg.

After fighting for years with my doctors over amputation, my foot miraculously improved. Tests for bacteria came back negative. There were no more fever or chills.

OH MY GOD.

What if I allowed them to cut my leg off below the knee? You can't glue it back on! It wouldn't grow back. After years of treatments, doctors, hospitals and all those expenses my foot was better!

Thank you, God.

When the Armstrongs returned to LA (from London), I was told the deal on the house fell through. They were back at square one. Not to worry though, they would find another.

The nanny already sanded the hardwood floors and Russell, himself, ripped out the living room fireplace mantel. My design assistants and I worked on their drawings for months. How could the deal fall apart at this point? It was inexplicable.

Years later, I learned the house was owned by an acquaintance who lent them the key so they could show it to me. They kept the key even though the deal wasn't consummated. The friend had no idea they moved into the house and tore it apart.

While working with the Armstrongs, I made the mistake of giving them a $45,000 personal check in exchange for more shares of My Medical Records Global, the start-up company I invested $50,000 in. Russell said another investor was ill and needed to redeem his shares assuring me this would pay off big time.

My check was made out to Russell's capital investment firm, not My Medical Records Global. He was handling the transaction and said it was no different than making my check out to Fidelity and instructing my broker to buy shares of Microsoft.

The "right" house in Beverly Hills never came along. They rented a home in Hollywood Hills. Taylor was cast in *Real Housewives of Beverly Hills* and Russell claimed to be opening a restaurant with Eva Langoria. Beso. When he told me he was the 51% owner, it sounded impressive, but I had my doubts.

After six years of marriage Taylor filed for divorce claiming she had been verbally and physically abused and couldn't take it anymore. That was shortly before she and Russell were named in a lawsuit claiming he misappropriated My Medical Records Global funds which she helped him spend.

Two weeks later Russell committed suicide leaving his wife responsible for the financial disaster he left behind. She had no money. Having no assets, the case settled out of court. Stressed out Taylor agreed to relinquish her 10-carat yellow diamond engagement ring valued at approximately $250,000 and several Hermes Birkin handbags which turned out to be fakes. Years afterwards the company went down the tubes along with my investment.

Jeff always said I was too gullible—the one tragic flaw with Leos.

SOUR
AND SWEET

In 2009 another doctor at Northwestern Memorial Hospital was experimenting with skin grafts for the diabetic foot. A healthy piece of skin removed from an area of one's body is used to hopefully remedy the foot dilemma. "The flap" includes skin and fat or skin, fat and muscle depending upon the circumstances. Dr. Giegerich said the results of several of his patients' having had this procedure were "encouraging".

He urged me to meet this doctor. I had nothing to lose except half my leg. Having tried every other options, I now became the subject of the bible verse *ye of little faith.*

Nonetheless, I made an appointment with the surgeon. Of course, he encouraged the operation and after my examination, said the skin, fat and muscle would come from my right thigh. The wound needed extra filling the muscle would provide.

I returned to the operating room on "get the flap" day.

Once awake, I commented to a nurse, "That was fast."

I was given heavy sedation before 6:00 am and the clock showed 6:30. She said she was glad I liked my nap; twelve and a half hours was a long time for the patient, surgeon and nurses. It was hard to be in shock only because I was still groggy. No one said this operation would take more time than my kidney transplant.

Afterwards, the pain was excruciating. There were many stitches and a long rut in my thigh after the doctor harvested the muscle from it.

New battle scars.

The next day, Ray Capitanini phoned. During surgery, I dreamt of Nada. Almost in tears Ray told me she died. His dear Nada, whom everyone loved and adored. Why her? She was a kind and gentle soul. I was in surgery for more than half a day—an awfully long surgery. I could have had a heart attack and gone to heaven. Or wherever. Why Nada I wondered?

I was discharged wearing that wound vac I continued to hate. I was ordered to wear it for two months. This doctor told me I must use crutches to promote healing.

He needed to come up with a new line.

Weekly visits to the surgeon's office continued for 10 months. Of course, things did not proceed as hoped. Eventually we needed to repeat the procedure. This time a piece of muscle was not used so the whole process went much faster and was far less painful. *Well, only a pain in my ass.*

***

"…when all else fails. art endures." Aunt Bea spoke from a podium in the Red Lacquer Ballroom at Chicago's historic Palmer House Hotel. The gilded interior with hand carved friezes was filled.

The occasion? Eighty-five-year-old Bea flew in from Palm Springs to present me with the Irv and Essee Kupcinet Leadership Award on behalf of the Chicago Academy for the Arts (CAA).

Overwhelmed? You bet. Not only at receiving the award but that my beloved, adopted, "Aunt" was the presenter. Even though she isn't really, she's family to me. Bea and I met in the late '80s when her luxurious Lake Shore Drive condominium flooded.

"It was love at first sight," we say of our meeting.

Bea Levi introduced me to the CAA shortly after we talked about water damage. Essee Kupcinet, her best friend and wife of Irv, late-night TV talk-show host, helped the school achieve recognition. Bea was recruited to charitably raise funds. She recalled Essee having her "begging, borrowing and practically stealing from everyone she could in the name of the Academy. Then, along came John Robert Wiltgen."

I was a willing co-conspirator and enthusiastic ambassador for the school. The arts always played a major role in my world. Bea reveled in tales of our joint fundraising efforts. When she invited me to the podium to accept the crystal award, I hobbled to the dais wearing my knee-high Cam Walker.

Not as polished as I would have liked.

Bea began to return to our table #1, but I insisted she re-join me. I would not accept the award unless I could share it with her. At 97½ she is still with us. She remembers everything. How much she pays her staff. How much her social security check is. Carol Channing's phone number even though Carol has been gone for several years now. Most of her friends have passed on, so I speak with her almost every day.

The next morning, I returned to the hospital for a second skip flap. Over time on the same crutches, with the same wound vac, it failed too. I wanted to fucking scream, but what good would it do?

And, quite frankly, I didn't have the energy.

It was hard work being optimistic. Three more design awards failed to lift my spirits. However, a phone call from actor, John Cusack, helped.

He wanted to make some changes to his new home, a 7,000 square foot Chicago condo. He was calling from the set of *2012*, a sci-fi film about the end of the world, in which he tries to save his family as everything falls apart.

I met John on crutches. He was sincere when he asked what happened. We sat down at his kitchen table with a spectacular view and talked about my foot and health in general for quite some time. His Mom was there. John was busy and shared his time with all of us. During our walk through his place (actually, I hobbled) he expressed dismay over how things failed to come together. John asked if I could come back the next day to continue our discussion. As a result, I worked with him for seven years doing, undoing, and redoing different rooms for him.

ME AND Mr. JONES

For years, I lived totally exhausted by the end of every day. Wearing a PICC line 3 months in then, 3 months out to give my body a rest, kept me at home most evenings in my bed watching my favorite cable station. On the weekends, I rarely got out of bed trying to regain strength trying to obey the doctor's orders of staying off my feet. So, I was home alone a good deal.

Jeff had a new boyfriend although he did visit and was always concerned about me. Jimmy had homes in LA, Palm Springs, Atlanta, Blue Ridge and Hawaii although he traveled more often to places where he didn't have them. It was hard to keep up with him. Consequently, I did not see him often.

Bored with TV, I started investigating assorted chat lines. Men. Women. It didn't matter. I had always been a good talker. Much to my delight, I conversed with people from all around the globe.

Late one Friday night I met someone with whom I had an instant fascination. It's strange isn't it? That you can get a feeling for someone through a computer.

Without exchanging our real names, I enjoyed our late-night conversations. He was witty and quick and charming. And smart. For all those reasons, I enjoyed his virtual company even though I had no idea what he even looked like. He was exceptionally private but asked all kinds of questions of me.

What did I do for work? Who did I work for? He didn't know much about the design world except what he saw on HGTV. I revealed my numerous episodes on that cable network and others. Was I married? Did I have children? Then he'd disappear without even a "goodbye".

The internet was our only contact. Sometimes I'd not hear from him for months. Not one word, so I chatted with other people. It was entertainment. Innocent. And then, like David Copperfield, he would reemerge.

Over time I learned about him. He was born in Chicago, the second of seven boys. When he was still young his family moved to Seattle. His maternal grandmother moved to the Pacific Northwest years earlier and said it offered many job opportunities. His mother packed the then 3 boys on a train and his family headed west. While there may have been a lot of job opportunities his dad didn't like to work. He was a mean, abusive alcoholic.

Later, he described his past as dark, filled with cruelty and unhappiness. When he graduated from high school his father gave him a suitcase. He packed it and moved back to Chicago to live with his grandmother who worked in a hospital. He got a job there, starting in the laundry department. Then, after going to night school, he became a respiratory therapist. Finally, a nurse. Pediatrics. Emergency room. ICU.

When I finally met Steven (yes, that was his real name), he worked as an intensive care nurse. His medical background made our connection intense. I disclosed my history to him. He was understanding and compassionate.

Eventually, I conjured up the nerve to question him about my suspicion.

"Are you married?"

Long pause. Then, "yes."

I thought so.

"What are you doing on-line?"

"It's complicated."

"Tell me..."

He had a family. A wife, a daughter, and a son. He loved them more than anything but was troubled he was no longer "in-love" with his wife. He needed to figure it out. For the past five or six years he thought maybe he developed a desire for men. He wasn't sure where these feelings came from. He was attracted to women, including his wife, but became drawn to men making him question his tendencies.

Was it just a fantasy of what sex with a man is like?

I understood. I told him I went through similar conflicts when I was much younger. I did not have a wife and/or kids. That certainly complicated things.

Steven was dealing with a lot of complex issues at home and did not feel like he could relinquish his responsibilities and so he stayed for several more years.

I was impressed with his sense of duty. I wish my father was like him.

It was almost a year before we finally agreed to meet. He came to my home. Not certain if I was a psychopathic serial killer, he gave my name and phone number to his best friend. Just in case. On the other hand, I didn't tell anyone anything.

He was blown away, not by me, but by my Egyptian Temple décor. He said he'd never seen anything like it, to which I replied, he must have missed that episode on HGTV.

With his salt and pepper hair and clean-shaven face he was a handsome devil. Tall. Built. Well groomed. Clean cut. Perfect manners. Perpetually tan in a natural way. Not like George Hamilton. More like a Viking Sun God.

Immediately, I felt comfortable around him. He dealt with the sickest patients in the hospital. For that reason, I trusted he might be able to deal with me and my permanently bandaged foot which was falling apart.

Slowly he revealed more details about his home life. He was so attached. So conflicted. I felt bad. Numerous times I told him we shouldn't see each other. It wasn't right. Coming from my own broken family, I felt terribly guilty.

Years later he quit his job at the hospital where he climbed his way up the ladder to a hospital administrator. It was time for a change. Steven took a job in the city working for a large insurance company.

During many of our Friday night visits, the one night each week he would come by after work, he watched me infuse different drugs through my PICC line and then fall asleep. If my home health care nurse visited me while he was there, he asked questions about my prognosis. Steven became an awesome friend. Sincere. Compassionate. Understanding. Devoted. He was wise and also extremely evolved spiritually.

One evening, as he was concocting dinner with the limited foodstuff in my frig, he referred to a presentation made to his department by a nurse from a suburban hospital. She promoted an innovative product that allegedly closed stubborn wounds by applying tissue created from the foreskin of a DNA perfect little boy considered to be a universal donor.

The hybrid tissue, grown in a lab, produced the equivalent of 4 football fields of the material. By providing living cells, proteins and collagen, it plays an active role in healing. When applied to a wound, the healing process begins within weeks. Steven hoped the procedure would help me.

New products and procedures are introduced to the world every day. I was so desperate to fix my foot I would have dipped it in lava oozing from a volcano if someone said it would solve my problems. Even if it gave me "Obsidian Foot" if that's a thing.

So, I went to yet another hospital every week for these hybrid tissue applications. Of course, after the first 8, there was minimal change. Doctors in the clinic said I needed another 8 sessions. Sadly, the results were no better. My brother Ray attended the 15th treatment with me. Steven could not go, and I am not sure we were at that point in our relationship. I needed someone smart who could be impartial to listen to the doctors. One said he would *now* begin to treat me as a "special case".

Ray and I looked at each other aghast. Why did they wait 15 weeks to seriously evaluate my situation? My confidence in them totally eroded. I felt misled. I was so pissed and worn out from all the experimental treatments I wanted to drive my car into the lake.

But I didn't. I just bought a newer BMW 7 series and I liked it too much.

Type 1 diabetes and I tackled one disaster after another. It can be a harsh lifestyle causing both physical and emotional devastation. Out of desperation, I embraced every new treatment hoping for even a shred of relief.

I was extremely optimistic when sealed in the glass-like coffin. The HBOT treatments provided no benefit other than supplying an extra two hours of sleep each day. I tried to remain positive about "the flap". I took a chance on skin grafts. Unfortunately, all I was doing was scheduling disappointments. However, no matter how difficult it was to remain hopeful, I refused to give up.

Another friend mentioned a prominent research surgeon at the University of Illinois Hospital who developed a "functional" cure for diabetes. This doctor pioneered transplanting human pancreatic islet cells eliminating the need for prescription insulin. Harvested from cadavers, transplanted cells stimulate the production of natural insulin and regulate glucose levels.

This is one of the most promising means to a cure for diabetes.

I met the innovative transplant surgeon bio-engineering professor, Jose Oberholzer, over lunch. The results of his clinical trials showed success in keeping a growing number of type 1 diabetics off prescription insulin for lengthy periods of time, some for a decade.

I wanted that to be me.

Oberholzer is enormously passionate about enabling people like me to live a non-diabetic life. About one-third of the human pancreatic cells harvested annually are suitable for use in his lab. Three are necessary for each islet-cell transplant. Oberholzer is also striving to develop an unlimited source of artificial islet cells for thousands of transplants and hoping to perfect an encapsulation process to eliminate the need for anti-rejection drugs.

After living with type 1 diabetes for many years, the doctor's accomplishments amazed me. I promoted his triumphs and future goals with everyone who crossed my path. Letters, phone calls, a blog, a press release. At a benefit Steven and I chaired for the Chicago Diabetes Project (which Oberholzer founded), patients spoke of how their lives returned to a state of normalcy they hadn't lived in years. With Oberholzer's encouragement, I decided to pursue the idea of such a transplant.

This procedure could eliminate my need for daily insulin and prevent many of the complications caused by diabetes. However, during the examination Dr. Oberholzer informed me I would need twice the amount of immunosuppressants to keep the islet cells functioning. The additional drugs would, most likely kill my mother's kidney within one year.

I would need another kidney transplant.

As much as I wanted to be cured of this enfeebling disease, I was not willing to risk killing her gift. Nor did I want to gamble further complications from an increased amount of anti-rejection drugs. My dream, to not be a diabetic, vanished.

Nonetheless, I still considered myself lucky. The interaction with the people I encountered every day distracted me and made me feel vital.

HIS EXCELLENCY

In October of 2004 Donald Trump purchased the Sun Times building on the Chicago River for $73 million. Every developer in Chicago passed on the opportunity saying no one of any means would ever move to *that* part of town. It wasn't Streeterville or the Gold Coast. But when Trump International Hotel and Tower was completed, closings on the sold luxury condominiums began and sales continued. The gleaming tower was three blocks from my office making JRWD the perfect choice of buyers needing professional design services with their new homes.

My friend Kiyoko was a sales agent for the luxurious development since the first day of presales. She introduced me to a client who expressed interest in 4,000 square feet of raw space on the 86th floor. That condominium had 12-foot ceilings with floor to ceiling windows and postcard-like views to the North and East.

Layers of family and friends represented the actual buyer. Two doctors interviewed me. Then, a nephew. All with African accents so thick it was difficult understanding their version of the King's English. When I passed their examinations, a time was set to meet "His Excellency". He was neither a king nor a member of a royal family, but he was extremely wealthy with homes in Maryland, Boston, New York City, London, a faraway place called Lagos and who knew where else. Plus, a "house" with wings (private jet) to transport him from one place to another.

Kiyoko and I met the Nigerians in Trump Tower's residential lobby. The sale was not consummated, but she was doing everything possible to make that happen including introducing me. Kiyoko knew I could design and build out the raw space exquisitely and furnish it to make it worthy of her billionaire client. The nephew, the doctors and a handful of other advisors were also present.

Contrary to our prior meetings, they were dressed in large, free flowing robes over shirt and trousers (more like pajama bottoms) with sandals. Each ensemble was more elegant than the other. Selling unique, unexpected style, I wore a made-to-order Tom Ford suit. When His Excellency entered the lobby, everyone, well not Kiyoko or I, dropped to their knees and kissed his sandaled feet.

"Do I have to do that?" I whispered to Kiyoko.

She looked up and smiled. "Not unless you want to."

"Well, not this time," I smiled back at her. "I haven't even met him yet."

She took me by the arm and said, "Let me make the introductions…"

Eight of us crammed into one of the elevators and went to the 86th floor. The Nigerians were conversing in a language that didn't come close to anything I'd ever heard before. There was a lot of laughing which I hoped was a good sign. When Kiyoko unlocked the door to the condominium, I took over walking them through rooms that didn't yet exist, holding up renderings to enable them to visualize an impeccably designed home.

I could have gone on and on trying to sell the condo with my services, but his Excellency raised his hand and announced I was his man. His friends had done their research and, after several other interviews, determined it would be me. He would purchase the raw space and directed me to follow up with his nephew, Fola. Then he left. His plane was waiting.

The project was finished in six months. That was record time to design, build, and furnish a four bedroom, four and one-half bath home in the demanding tower that didn't allow workmen to make noise before 10 am and had to leave the premises by 4:30 pm. Everyone in my office worked around the clock and on weekends making certain contracts were reviewed and tradesmen showed up on site when needed. This home had to reflect the very best of John Robert Wiltgen Design. I knew it could buy us other opportunities in the building and there were plenty to be had with 485 residences, most of them with curved walls and large round concrete columns.

When I finally retired, I had 27 homes in the extravagant tower to my credit.

While still a work in progress, a major shelter magazine committed to featuring this project as their first editorial about Trump Tower Chicago living.

My client was impressed we finished so quickly. After our first meeting I spoke with him personally only twice. Quickly earning his trust, he told me to "just do it." I did. So, he flew in from somewhere to see it. He was excited.

The powder room featured a wall mounted sink floating on a mirrored wall. The great room was organized with four seating areas covered in ivory leather. Each area was designed to accommodate a different number of guests. A combination of mid-century modern and contemporary furnishings was chosen to compliment the building's architecture. In a second powder room, we installed a backlit agate mirror frame and matching vanity top. A modern Murano glass chandelier in the dining room came from the same manufacturer that has been supplying the Vatican for the past 400 years. The stainless-steel dining table base supports a bull horn veneer top. The kitchen is a blend of white lacquer and African mahogany cabinetry. The gracious master bedroom includes a piece of artwork installed on the wall above the king size bed. It is so big it would not fit into the gigantic freight elevator. The frame broke as the movers tried manipulating it. Nonetheless, they brought it up and we reframed it inside the residence.

Upon completion of the tour, His Excellency smiled saying he loved it all. I knew he was impressed when he immediately asked me to design another project for him. He wanted a new house in Lagos, Nigeria.

AFRICA.

Could I prepare a complete set of architectural drawings as well as select all the interior finishes, furniture, and artwork? Of course, I could. I just did that for him.

My head was spinning. This would be the most substantial commission of my career. I was going to Lagos to design an estate from the ground up for the Asiwaju (leader). Bola Ahmed Adekunle Tinubu could have anyone in the world and he commissioned ME.

UNDER
AFRICAN SKIES

Our first trip to Lagos was in August 2010. Ray and I traveled from O'Hare International Airport to JFK where we were meeting Fola who was coming from Washington, DC. Together, the three of us were going to Nigeria.

When it was time to board, Fola was nowhere in sight. Not knowing what else to do, we left the lounge and headed toward the plane. Hopefully, he was there.

Once seated, my phone rang.

"Fola?"

"Yeah, John. Where are you?" It was his deep King's English laced with a thick Nigerian dialect.

"We're on the plane," I told him scanning the front cabin with admiration. "They just started boarding. Where…"

"You have to get off!" he interrupted.

"What?" He was kidding, right?

"My train was late, and I will not make it through security to arrive at the gate on time…"

I could not believe it.

"…and it is not safe for you and Ray to go there without me."
The phone went dead.

Ray looked at me questioningly. "Was that Fola?"

"No, it was the milkman."

"What did he say?"

"He said they are out of skim milk; they only have 2%. And get off the plane. He is not going to make it and it is not safe for us to go there without him."

"Whaaaat?" Ray questioned in utter disbelief.

I shook my head. "I wish I was kidding. No skim milk. Come on let's go…" I put on my sport coat, grabbed my carry-on bags and headed for the door.

Never one to waste time, Ray already spread his computer and papers out in his secluded booth. And he befriended the flight attendants working our cabin and felt the need to say buh-bye.

That was how our first trip to Nigeria began. We arrived three days later. Arik Airplanes do not travel from JFK daily. As we quickly learned, they fly every OTHER or every third day. The same plane travels back and forth and needs maintenance to keep its wings attached. And gas.

As soon as I sat down in my station, I fell asleep. When the flight attendant awakened me for breakfast, I felt refreshed and ready to conquer another world. I lifted the window shade and saw land. We were almost 6,000 miles from home. Mom, Steven and my doctors all thought I was crazy traveling to Africa. And maybe I was, but I craved the excitement.

My foot was sealed in "the boot". The sore on the bottom never healed. Twelve effen years of cleaning it, wrapping my foot with bandages and sterile gauze. Plus, all the PICC lines and antibiotics. Thank God I was escaping my real world and beginning a new adventure. I refused to let my foot and all my other problems stop me.

Sometime during the flight, Fola changed his suit and shirt for an agbada, those three articles of clothing everyone but Kiyoko and I wore in the lobby of Trump Tower when I first met my client. The ensemble is a status symbol in Nigeria. Fola's had French cuffs and was made of the most luxurious blue cotton fabric. Proudly, he paraded off the plane.

The air was hot and muggy. I wished Ray and I wore agbadas too. They were loose and airy, perfect for the equatorial weather, not like our belted trousers, button down shirts, and sport coats.

Some of the 512 distinctly different Nigerian languages spoken that day must have been music to someone's ears. Not mine but someone's. English is the official language but His Excellency (that is how I address the former governor of Lagos State) and his friends speak Yoruba when they do not want Ray or me to know what they are saying.

Don't lose sight of Fola I kept telling myself as he pointed to a line for visitors without Nigerian passports. A uniformed man ordered Ray and me to get in line, single file. Collectively we moved slowly. When it was finally our turns, Ray and I were ushered to separate windows.

"Why are you here?" Not even a good afternoon, sir.

"Business," I replied with a smile.

"Which oil company?" assumed the customs officer.

"I am not with an oil company," I responded as calmly as possible. With my six-month Nigerian Visa, I didn't expect to be questioned.

"What are you doing here, then?" he demanded.

"I am designing a private estate…"

"What?"

"For the Asiwaju…" I used my client's title bestowed upon him by the King.

His eyes nearly popped from his head, their huge whites contrasting sharply with his dusky skin tones. He quickly stamped my passport and waved me on. I jerked my way through the crowd to reach my brother. As we continued with the masses, Fola appeared accompanied by two guards carrying AK47's.

"Welcome to Lagos," he exclaimed with a huge grin on his black as night face.

Lagos is much like any other metropolis. Because of the immense population, the streets and sidewalks are more crowded than most American cities. The only difference is it is much easier to find someone grilling a pig on the sidewalk in front of a bank there, than the streets of NYC.

Almost 40 percent of the Nigerian population live beneath the poverty level, surviving on an average equivalent of less than $2 US per day. Many live in Makoko, a slum consisting of connected boats, pontoons and one-room homes on stilts in a murky swamp beneath Africa's longest bridge near the airport.

Nigeria's middle class, who make up about 34 percent of the population, include entry level attorneys, bankers and accountants earning about $800 US/month. My Lagos lawyer is not entry level as her hourly rate is the equivalent of $400 US. The salary of a newly licensed doctor at a private hospital starts at about $1,000 a month. A single person, who is not an expat, can live comfortably on that income. Expats living in guarded, gated, communities with private schools pay considerably more to reside there.

The city's upper class consists mostly of business moguls and politicians. Some households earn the equivalent of $1 M US annually. And much more. For these fortunate families, there are country clubs, shopping malls, designer clothing, fabulous jewelry, trendy restaurants, hip nightclubs, condominium towers, houses, nice houses and even nicer houses. A lot like America.

Nigeria has many daily headaches, but power is by far the worst. It constantly failed in our luxury hotel. Not only our hotel and the island, but throughout all of Lagos—Africa's largest city with its metropolitan population of 15.3 million. That is 2 times as many people as NYC. Less than half of Lagos citizens are fortunate enough to have electricity.

Our hotel rooms were carpeted wall-to-wall and fragranced with bug spray. Was that a sign? I wondered if the place was infested, and management was trying to eliminate insects we prayed we'd never see. Are they big? Do they bite? Could they be poisonous? These are things we do not think about while tucked beneath our 610-thread count Egyptian cotton sheets back home.

Ray and I had connecting rooms in case I had a "problem". Before we left, he checked out hospitals in Lagos and learned that anyone of means who requires serious medical treatment is usually evacuated by air to a country with better facilities. He signed us both up for comprehensive medical insurance including provisions for international medical transport. If needed we would be taken to Frankfurt or Rome, not Monte Carlo or St. Tropez as I hoped.

The day after our arrival Fola, Ray and I were driven to the site where my client's estate would be built. None of us "DEETed" that morning with the insect repellent used to deter mosquitos. However, we were taking Malarone, a tablet which prevents the dangerous blood disease.

Nigeria is a malaria hotbed accounting for up to 25 percent of the cases worldwide. To make matters worse, we arrived as the first rainy season of the year ended and the newest batch of mosquitos hatched.

The location was a mess. Overgrown grounds. Landscape in shambles. Two houses. Fola smiled and urged us out of the car to inspect and photograph the area. The ground was wet. Some areas had muddy ponds which were breeding grounds for the Anopheles mosquito. I didn't want to appear chicken…

Ray got out of the BMW. And Fola got out. So, I HAD to get out. Ray, the designated photographer with the expensive camera, began taking pictures of everything. Good. The sooner he obtained the photos we needed, the sooner we could get back in the car.

The existing houses were worthless. They were deserted and literally falling apart. It wouldn't take much to tear them down. No need to go inside which reduced our chances of stepping into a nest of West African carpet vipers accounting for 90 percent of the snake bites in Nigeria and 60 percent of human snakebite fatalities. Despite their smaller size (approximately 20″ when full grown) their hemotoxic venom makes them one of the world's most dangerous snakes.

When we finished, I was sweating like a pig, which was a good thing because pigs are immune to snakebites. Farmers in Nigeria raise them to clear their land of the poisonous serpents.

The two-acre site was on Ikoyi, Lagos's most affluent island with the tightest density of millionaires in the city and most expensive real estate on the African continent. I was expected to transform the mess into a luxurious and secure estate.

The schedule called for completion of a full set of drawings within three months. We had just begun to analyze how each of the buildings would fit into the lay of the land. The Israeli general contractor needed foundation plans. Pages and pages of construction drawings with a great number of details. Electrical. Plumbing. Interior elevations. Sections of a three-story library, two-story atrium, two separate stair halls, and glass enclosed elevator. They asked for a mosque which would be used by the men and Christian chapel for the women. And 3-D color renderings to illustrate the finished appearance of the gardens, exteriors, and interiors of the estate.

The grounds required guard houses; one at the main entrance with an attached conference center for the convenience of those permitted an audience with His Excellency but denied access to the main house. Another at the service entrance. A water tank, purification center and building for the generator also had to be located somewhere. Plus, we needed a 10,000-gallon diesel fuel tank buried underground.

This was a bigger than life puzzle. Could I get all the pieces to fit together?

There was also a long list of security issues. The grounds were divided into undetectable sections. Guards could not co-mingle with others outside of their assigned area. If they did, they would be shot. And bullet proof glass of course, but for what caliber gun? That was the question.

From there we explored Ikoyi. Manicured lawns with amazing flowers and tall, elegant Nigerian palms create a fertile picture of an opulent lifestyle. Well paved roads without potholes differentiate this district from the rest of Lagos.

One evening Fola took us to dinner at a fashionable restaurant on the lagoon. We met the Honorable Prince Adesegun Abiodun Oniru, the Commissioner for Waterfront Infrastructure and oldest son of Oba Idowu Oniru of Iruland.

Nigerians are obsessed with titles. They flaunt flamboyant names. Fola presented my brother as Engineer Raymond Thomas Wiltgen III and me as International Award-Winning Designer John Robert Wiltgen, professional member of the International Interior Design Association. That was a mouthful.

The prince was impressed we were imported from Chicago to work on His Excellency's project and invited us to see his land development with its solar-powered streetlights. When I said we'd love to, the prince smiled, suggested a date to us and stood. Men at another table rose and guarded the royal as they escorted him down the dock to his beautiful, gold and burgundy, 50-foot Cigarette Marauder with three 800 HP supercharged engines providing a cruising speed of up to 85 MPH.

As they roared away, I thought, "I could get used to this…"

Despite the similarities to NYC or Chicago, there were also many differences. The culture of Lagos was not the same. I had so much to learn and so little time. But I do love a good challenge. That's what keeps me going.

Totally unrelated to my client's estate, Fola introduced Ray and me to two men developing a 27-hole golf course community. They envisioned it as a PGA Championship members only club.

The site is on vacant shores of the Atlantic Ocean blessed with colossal surf and stately Palm trees kissed by a glorious breeze. But the site improvements stopped. A tribe lived on part of this land for hundreds of years and they had no intention of leaving.

But that wasn't why the developers needed our help. The architectural plan showed both members and staff entering the clubhouse through the same doors. And there were no service roads to either the clubhouse, proposed beachside hotel or beach, so members who had paid an exorbitant amount, hotel guests, and workers would all use the same private road. Was there an opportunity of working on this project too? It was exciting.

Another day, Fola announced a visit to the current home of his uncle, my client.

Staring from the window of our chauffeur-driven BMW, I was always looking out the window. Poorer citizens ride on motorcycle taxis while commuting to work. Holding on for dear life, someone sits on the handlebars while the driver looks around that passenger to see where they are going. One or two more passengers sit on the back of the seat. It's like a magic trick. Occasionally a passenger has a kitchen sink above his or her head loaded with two bags of groceries. No helmets. A church bus ran into one of these taxis and just kept going.

My client's home is surrounded by a red brick wall so high it's impossible to see what's on the other side. Lots of razor wire crowns the top. It must be an extremely lucrative business in Lagos as it is everywhere. At one end of the wall is a black, solid iron gate and guard house.

Our driver spoke to an armed guard. Three more opened the gate for us.

Inside was an enormous parking lot filled with Mercedes, BMWs, SUV's and a trophy Rolls Royce. Cars are like flowers in Nigeria and a garden of cars, of course, a status symbol.

The exterior of the house looked almost Brutalist. Massive, somewhat fortress-like. A turret with an octagon shaped roof. Little windows. Not what I expected.

Through the screen door were more uniformed guards. A metal detector. Fola made some sort of humorous remark to them in Yoruba as we were ushered through. Once the guards stopped laughing, patted us down and searched Ray's briefcase, Fola gestured us to follow him.

The dark living room had low ceilings and traditional window treatments because heavy damask fabric and a crowd of people block out the sunlight. Men, women, and children were seated everywhere, even on the floor.

Fola led us to another room, empty and air conditioned. Thank God. Or Allah. Whomever.

"My uncle has a few appointments before us," Fola stated. "It shouldn't be too long."

The ceramic tile floor and overstuffed leather furniture was nothing as impressive as what I designed for their Trump Tower home. An exposed cord powered a wall-mounted TV. There was another TV on a stand. More cords. It was a man-cave appearing to have been created without professional help. Fola told me a designer from the UK was involved. For the first time he was not smiling.

"This is one of the private waiting rooms," Fola declared. "More like a VIP lounge," he laughed.

"Who are all those people out there?" I inquired.

"People come to see my uncle whenever he is here," he said. "They come to thank him for a favor OR ask for a favor OR want him to settle a dispute." He shrugged his shoulders and continued smiling.

There was a knock on the door. So soon? Wrong. It was a young woman asking if we wanted anything. She spoke to Fola in Yoruba.

"It is going to be a while," Fola advised.

"How long?" Ray asked.

Fola shrugged his shoulders again still smiling, "I don't know..."

Fola had a pocket full of cell phones in his agbada. He returned to his constant texting on three or four of them. Ray pulled out his laptop, so did I. Six hours and a few candy bars later His Excellency came through the door.

And that is a short waiting period. People often hold out two or three times longer for an audience with the Asiwaju.

He and his wife live on the second floor. When Madame wants a cup of coffee she dresses, saunters down the stairs, greets 20 or 30 strangers, before reaching the kitchen. Pretending not to be important, she goes to the kitchen herself instead of sending a staff member. Her bearing is regal, and she's always elegantly dressed. There are guards everywhere. When she saw me, her face lit up.

"John, what are you doing here?" asked the model-like woman who turns heads whether at home or traveling internationally.

She wore a bright yellow geles, a gravity-defying headwrap favored by Nigerian women, and a floral-print wrap dress with sleeves cut around colorful flowers. While in her native country, she is the personification of the traditional Nigerian wife.

I filled her in on our trip.

She had never met Ray, so I introduced them.

"You are John's brother?" she asked.

He nodded. "Have been for almost 50 years now."

She eyed him up and down. We don't look alike, and he could have been joking.

"When are you two going home?"

"Sunday evening," I answered.

"Then you must come back for brunch," she declared. "I will prepare a sumptuous feast for you before you leave."

A sumptuous feast? We had been so careful about the food we ate. What would we do if she served something that made us sick on the plane 10 hours later? Or, if I ingested a tape worm that grew 26 feet long inside my intestines? But I reminded myself, we were invited by the wife of the former governor of Lagos State and one of the most powerful men in all of Africa. She too was powerful in her own right and became a Nigerian senator.

"Thank you," I replied. "That is very kind of you. What time should we be here?"

The rest of the week passed quickly. Sunday came before we knew it. Regretfully, we were leaving. Finding this world so intriguing, I didn't want to go home. Yet.

Sunday morning our car, driver and bodyguard were waiting for us outside our hotel to take us to His Excellency's home.

We wore suits to brunch. Though we were both measured for agbadas, they were not yet finished by the tailor.

His Excellency was in London on business, so the house was nearly empty. The usual crowd waiting to get their minute or two with him was absent. It was just a bunch of bodyguards, our hostess, Ray and me.

Madame Oluremi (called Remi) Tinubu greeted us graciously. The youngest of 12 children, she has degrees in botany and zoology. Again, she wore an amazing Nigerian wrap dress. Another floral print, remarkably chic and, as before, culturally appropriate. I will forever be curious about how her headdress is tied two feet above her. However, her jewelry was the most amazing detail of her ensemble.

She wore a magnificent breastplate of cabochon rubies mixed with round cut pink diamonds set in platinum with matching earrings, a bracelet, and a big chunky ring. I could not stop staring. I had never seen anything like this. And it was only brunch. What does she wear to dinner?

The faux traditional dining table, probably made in China, was filled with an assortment of Nigerian dishes. Most were cooked like the Isi Ewe, a recipe requiring at least one goat head. It is seasoned with Tazi leaf and Euro seeds. The pepper soup is made with pepper. And snail's kabob - a sumptuous and crunchy dish - leaves one with a rewarding feeling which they say often leads to sex. Some of the food was raw including a beautiful vegetable salad and brightly colored fruit sticks.

I waited for Madame to be seated. Her fine bone china and brilliant cut crystal were elegant. Water glasses. Wine glasses. Champagne flutes. Did she dine like this every day?

We made small talk…

How were the kids? Her two daughters. When was she returning to Chicago? Was Ray married? Did he have children? Two brothers who worked together—that was nice. What did we think of her country? The new house was going to be much larger than she wanted. She did not like the idea of a big house. But she would like a pool not out in the open so her husband's visitors could not see her. She doesn't use their pool now as everyone can see her.

OKAY. Good to know. Brunch was more productive than I expected. I continued listening.

At one point, she noticed I was not sampling any of the salads or berries on the table. "John, why are you not having some salad? And the berries are so fresh—they are delicious. Enjoy them."

I didn't know what to say. I did not want her to think us rude.

Then she laughed. "Are you afraid you are going to get sick? Do not worry. We have a water filtration system here. Everyone does. The food will not make you ill. Trust me."

So, we chowed down on the salad and berries and did not get sick then or on subsequent trips. After that we ate everything and never had a tape worm. Or malaria.

Our parting conversation went something like this….

"So, when are the two brothers leaving?"

"Our Arik Airplane is scheduled to take off at midnight. But they are not too punctual."

She nodded. "Nonetheless, you should leave the hotel around 8:30. It could take an hour."

"We are packed. We just need to go back and shower, change our clothes, check out…"

"I will send a police escort."

I thanked her profusely. We hugged goodbye. I wasn't sure if that was appropriate, her being the former First Lady of Lagos State in Nigeria, Africa. But she was procuring a police escort for us which I hoped wasn't necessary. It seemed like we were getting close.

As we exited through the metal detector, she followed us out and waved goodbye. Leaving the empty courtyard, her diamond breastplate glistened in the afternoon African sun. I turned around and waved goodbye.

Oluremi is a goddess. The gates closed behind us and we were gone. I was sad. In a short time, I became quite fond of Lagos and its people. We were going home, and I wondered if we would ever return.

AFRICAN REGGAE

But we did return.

With Brent crude oil prices averaging almost $80.00 per barrel and continuing to rise, Fola, Ray, Susan (Tjarksen) and I were forming our own real estate development company—Atlantic Coast Development Resources—in Lagos. Nigeria was then the fifth largest supplier of oil to the US and its economy was booming. The U.S. Dept. of State warned American citizens of the risks of travel to Nigeria, recommending we avoid all but essential trips.

Were we crazy or what?

The previous day, Ray—the smart one in our family—closed on the purchase of his newest business—nuts. He was going into the nut manufacturing business. Not the edible kind. Ray's nuts are a patented, vibration-resistant type used on railroad and mining cart ties that don't require regular tightening. Designed to save his customers buckets of money he wouldn't be making bolts, just the nuts.

After the closing, Ray phoned the U.S. Dept. of State advising its officials, despite their warnings, we were Lagos-bound. He bought travel insurance for us and went home to pack. Gail, his wife, was troubled. Once again, he was off to Africa. It's a long trip. Far from home. DANGEROUS so the State Department says. And he was going for my benefit.

Because of all my medical issues, I rarely traveled alone anymore. Certainly not when trekking 6,000 miles from home.

Ray is exactly what brothers are for.

Our flight was scheduled to leave at 11:00 pm and though we boarded on time, lift off didn't happen for 5 hours. Lagos is an 11½ hour flight from JFK. Since we were the only First-Class passengers, we were able to sit wherever we wanted.

Once the seat belt light went off somewhere over the Atlantic, Susan and I went to the bar. Our plane was a custom Airbus 340 with a full-service bar meaning it came with a bartender. It made the lengthy voyage fun. Perched on a chrome and ivory leather barstool, Susan ordered a glass of wine. I had my usual, a Diet Coke on ice. Three's my limit. We were the only ones there, so I consumed all the appetizers. Why does carb laden food taste so good?

Dinner was our first meal on the plane even though it was close to 6:30 am. I ordered Nigerian Pepper Soup, a mixed salad, and roasted chicken with fresh sautéed vegetables. Susan had the soup, salad and a fish entrée. For dessert, I took a Flurazepam. I keep a bottle in the pharmacy that always travels with me. I convinced Susan to take one too. Told her she would sleep like a baby.

After dinner Susan changed into her blue Arik Air pajamas. I slept in my street clothes because I was wearing the boot which makes it hard to take my pants off. Impossible for me to do in a tiny airplane bathroom. Even though we were conversing about sweet little nothings I was out the minute my head hit the pillow. I can sleep almost anywhere. Because I snore, she moved to another cubicle, far enough away not to be disturbed which was tricky, because Ray and Fola snore, too.

Sometime later a flight attendant awakened her with the news her husband (moi) was sick. She rushed to my bed shocked to find me convulsing. My eyes rolled into the back of my head, my tongue hung out and I shook like a wild man. Without delay, she straddled me and yelled, summoning someone to bring orange juice or a Coke. Regular, not diet. While waiting, she chewed on a piece of candy and then started French kissing me to get the candy into my mouth. I was too far gone to remember any of it. From past incidents Susan knew I couldn't chew anything. She was afraid I might choke on something hard or solid, maybe even bite off my tongue.

When I finally came to, I was soaking wet. Susan told the crew I choked on a chicken bone from dinner. That is how the staff filled out the official paperwork required whenever there is an airborne medical incident of consequence. My blood glucose level probably dropped to 10 or 12. I did not want Fola to know I am a diabetic since childhood, at least not until the contract for my client's estate was signed and the development corporation was a done deal. For the remainder of the flight Susan slept with me, one hand on my chest making sure I was still breathing.

She whispered in my ear, "I love you, Johnny."

Susan is the only one allowed to call me that. My Mother doesn't even call me Johnny. Everything was good. But I scared the shit out of her, leaving her wondering "WTF was I thinking when I agreed to go on this trip?"

MORE
AFRICAN REGGAE

As our plane touched down at Murtala Muhammed International Airport, Fola had us off and running. He said the King expected us. We checked into our hotel and were allowed a few scant minutes to freshen up. Unpacking and a shower had to wait.

Susan's tired eyes grew alert. She had no idea she would meet the incumbent "Oba" of Lagos of the Yoruba tribe in contemporary West Africa.

On May 23, 2003, Rilwan Babatunde Osuolale Aremu Akiolu was selected by oracles of the Lagos traditional kingdom who spoke with the gods. In a world of computers, technology and Ancestory.com, the King was made by traditional kingmakers. He was also confirmed by the Lagos State government.

As I quickly rummaged through my carry on stuffed with pharmaceuticals, there was a knock at the door. "The Oba?" a flabbergasted Susan asked. "What should I wear?"

"I hope that in the three suitcases you checked and the two you carried on, there's a dress and heels," I replied.

She had a classic little black dress. "It's short. That's all I brought in the dress department. I wanted to buy some authentic clothing here..."

"It will be fine," I said. "What about shoes?"

"I have the Stuart Weitzman pumps you bought me," she said, with a look that could sour lemons. She was totally dumbfounded—quite the attitude change for the ever-in-command dominatrix. Susan was afraid the shoes might be a tad too sexy for the king's court.

"They'll be perfect," I smiled. I liked the "tad too sexy" thing. That's why I bought them for her. Susan is a sex kitten.

Sounding like Mom, she asked if I needed something to eat before departing on the royal excursion.

"No. I just tested my sugar. I'm fine..."

You're sure? I'll bring the crackers," she schlepped a crate of crackers with peanut butter just in case...

"Okay." Whatever. "Let's go."

The official residence of the Oba, since 1705, is Iga Idungaran Palace. That's where we were headed. The palace was built by the Portuguese and presented as a gift to the then King. The grounds were first used to plant pepper. The name Pepper Palace is how Iga Idungaran translates. Some of the buildings in the "hood" were missing doors, windows, siding. Children were partially clothed. Everything was falling apart. A man was peeing in the street in front of the gods and everyone. But the bright colors of the traditional African garb worn by both men and women softened their poverty.

The 300+ year-old palace has undergone renovations. The compound is a haphazard mixture of colonial and modern styles. In 2007, the pure colonial architecture of the small castle was modernized. Residents adjacent to the palace were quietly moved as the monarch's "people" demolished their homes. They were razed to give rise to a 10-story tower serving as personal living quarters for the king, his wives and their children. The dead bodies of former Obas did not move with them. They are buried in assorted chambers throughout the original palace except the throne room which is reserved for the living monarch.

BTW. In case you are interested...tourists need to get permission before visiting the palace. Although there is really no such thing as tourism in Nigeria.

Less than two hours after landing we arrived at Iga Idungaran. The meeting held no urgency for the king. It was Fola's eagerness to present us, his trophy business partners, to the monarch. Importing a group of Americans to Lagos to start a real estate enterprise was a huge endorsement of Fola's dubious history of business successes. His Royal Majesty was to be impressed.

A portly, barefoot guard carrying an AK 47 (everyone has one) allowed us to enter. The reception area was filled with newspaper clippings, photographs and paintings of HRM. Many were gifts from friends and those wishing to endear themselves to the royal family. Memorabilia was scattered about the floor.

We were guided up a gracious but modern circular staircase to a second floor VIP waiting room. I was intrigued. When Ray and I had been here before we were not invited to climb these stairs. To my dismay it was furnished with the same dreadful leather furniture every local seemed to own.

Note to self: Speak to HRM about sprucing up his palatial digs with worthier furniture.

We were fascinated by more paintings of the Oba lining the walls. They were framed in heavily carved gold moldings—gold paint not gold leaf. One of them attempted to resemble *Napoleon Crossing the Alps*, a famous equestrian portrait by Jacques-Louis David. Only Napoleon wasn't on the horse, the Oba was.

I informed Susan about the sequestered space on the ground floor where high priests groomed the king prior to his coronation during a 91-day season of prayers and rituals to ensure his long and prosperous life. On our last visit, I asked HRM if I could see the space, but he diplomatically refused explaining that for centuries, only the man who would be king and his priests entered the consecrated chamber.

Suddenly, and without warning, a pair of doors were flung open by two more beefy, barefoot attendants. Staring directly at Susan, they announced "His Majesty will see you now..."

A rustic dais held a carved, wooden throne clad with animal hides. There sat the King. Considered one of Nigeria's most stylish, powerful and wealthy Obas, he was wearing a soiled Nike jogging suit that had been white once upon a time. He too, was barefoot and his toenails curled. They had not been trimmed in years. Next to him was a taxidermized lion.

Eyeing Susan, a smile lit his face. He beckoned to her, pointing to the chair nearest his throne.

She leaned ever so slightly to me and asked, ventriloquist-fashion, "What should I do?"

"Uhm, I think you should sit next to His Majesty," I replied. I wasn't good at ventriloquism.

As she nervously strutted her stuff to the chair the King indicated, Fola sunk his massive body reverently to his knees, hands on the ground in a bow before the Oba. Never have I seen him move so fast. Ray, a confirmed "When in Rome" kind of guy, followed suit. I tried too but stumbled and fell because the Cam Walker kept me off balance. Ray quickly righted me. On our hands and knees, it was hard not to notice Susan wasn't wearing underwear.

Gazing admiringly at her, the King continued smiling before speaking Yoruba to one of his attendants.

The imperial assistant addressed us in English. "On behalf of His Royal Majesty I would like to welcome the King's guests from America to Lagos. Nigeria is friends with America and the Oba of Lagos, Oba Rilwan Aremu Akiolu, is honored to receive our friends here at Iga Idungaran."

The greeting continued for some time. When the interpreter finished, I wondered who he thought we were. None of us were ambassadors or high-ranking government officials.

Speaking through his attendants the Oba told Susan he had several wives but none with blue eyes or blonde hair. He stared intently.

We laughed at HRM's translated sense of humor not then knowing he was a certified polygamist. The Nigeria Sun News quoted the ruler in an interview proclaiming any man who says he can do with just one wife deceives himself. The Oba had given hint of his desire to add more women to his harem. Our timing was perfect.

After the King dictated something to his assistant, a statement that went on and on, we were promptly dismissed. We nodded as if in China and thanked HRM profusely.

Back at the car Susan asked Fola what took place in the throne room. He said she was just married to His Royal Majesty!

"If I knew I was getting married, I'd have worn underwear," she quipped. We all laughed.

Fola told her not to worry. Wives of the king are often given gifts. Nice cars—a Bentley, Rolls Royce, even a Ferrari. Or a multi-million-dollar condominium on Banana Island or, even better, in London. And sometimes, a successful money-making business so they wouldn't have to ask the Oba for Naira.

Our days were filled with meetings as Fola continued to present us to an array of powerful business associates and politicians. At the end of our days, we usually met in one of our three hotel rooms to determine what was said at them. Their English was so thick we each came up with a different understanding.

One evening Fola announced we were going to Ghana the next morning and requested our passports. We needed visas which usually took 6 weeks. Ray and I handed ours over.

Another adventure.

Susan refused to relinquish hers. She was scared. The State department, her fiancé, probably Mom, and countless others cautioned her to keep her passport on her person. Ray asked if she wanted to stay behind in Lagos alone.

"No," she said with a "deer in headlights" look.

"Then give him your passport," RELUCTANTLY, I mean EXTREMELY RELUCTANTLY, she handed it to Fola. He quickly disappeared.

After a buffet dinner, Fola returned saying we needed professional head shots. Sometime after 11 pm, he drove us to a dark, dank, part of the city beneath a bridge in a crowded no man's land. Making our way through large groups of homeless-looking people, all I could think of was without passports we could easily be snuffed out and made to disappear. No problem.

The photo studio was impossible to find unless you'd been there before. There were no signs. The building was more like a hut. It had a dirty mattress on the ground and photos of scantily clad women thumb-tacked to the walls. I would not be able to run with the clunky boot, but Ray and Susan could. I hoped they would make it out of this menacing abyss alive.

Scary as it then seemed, probably because I've seen way too many action thrillers, the photographer was legit. He took our pics, disappeared for twenty minutes, and returned with a handful of printed color images. We looked awful. Maybe landscapes were his thing.

We flew on His Excellency's private jet. Susan sat in H E's seat scribbling a note to him on the outside of a box of Good 'N Plenty. Ray was up front with the pilot for part of the ride. A blonde Swedish flight attendant with a lovely accent and nice legs served us.

As we approached the airport in Accra, the control tower operator reported having no record of our flight plan. Our pilots told Ray it was filed before take-off, but this was the Ghanaians way of charging more money to land. Everything in Africa is about money and how much people have to throw around.

Our first stop was in the city of Accra to look at some acreage next to a shopping mall. His Excellency wanted our professional opinion of its potential and an estimate of how much it would cost. The lot was surrounded by a stone wall approximately five feet high, so we had to climb up for a serious look. On my way, I scraped my leg, ripped my pants, and started bleeding profusely. I mean really bleeding and they were the only pants I brought with me. We planned on staying overnight, maybe a total of 36 hours including airtime. Ray took out his Boy Scout first-aid kit, cleaned my gash, sprayed it with antiseptic and wrapped it with gauze. Everyone was afraid it would become infected. It was my left leg which still had osteomyelitis and cellulitis.

When we were done, we left Accra for the remote countryside to assess another property; a run-down hotel in the middle of the jungle. Susan rode in a separate SUV with Fola and some guards. Ray and I were in the other vehicle. It was the first time I worried about all of us. We were separated and I had no idea what was happening. I tried texting Susan repeatedly, but there was no answer making me worry more. Horrible thoughts crossed my mind. Again, I have seen too many action thrillers. I imagined the guys forcing themselves on her as we drove farther into the jungle. Then I thought of our machine gun-carrying guards ordering Ray and me to strip and run naked through the jungle, defenseless from the crocodile monitor (the longest known lizard in the world) or a 15-foot African Rock Python. My blood pressure soared.

It took about an hour and a half to reach our destination; a collection of powerless buildings, some with running water amid the jungle. Susan was fine. There was a wok on the floor of the restaurant's filthy open-aired kitchen. Instead, we ate peanut butter crackers.

On our way back to the city the driver instructed me to keep the tinted window closed. The guard did not want locals to know their passengers were Americans. "Could be dangerous" he said. We had a police escort, but our motorcycle cop wiped out in the middle of the road while literally "kicking" a moving car out of our way. He picked himself up and waived us on. Our driver continued without a second thought.

The next morning, after checking out, Fola announced we were going to meet the Vice President.

"Of what company?" I asked thinking he was with some real estate development firm.

"The Vice President of Ghana," he replied as if it was no big deal.

"What?" How about some warning so we would have packed better clothes? I had a fresh white button-down shirt but only my torn bloody pants. I needed to go shopping. Fast.

There wasn't enough time to go to the mall. One of the guards escorted Susan and me down the street. In one of the "retail" huts on a sidewalk, I spotted a stack of blue jeans. We entered. There was barely room for Susan, me, and the shop keeper. The guard waited outside.

"Can I help you?" the Ghanaian asked in more of the same heavily accented English.

"I need a pair of pants," I replied pointing to the tear outlined in blood.

"Yes sir. I can see that sir," he said, wrapping a cloth measuring tape around my waste. "34."

"I am not a 34," I protested.

"Yes, sir" he looked at the tape, "34."

He pulled a pair of jeans from a stack. I'll show him I thought. There was no dressing room. I turned around meaning anyone on the street would get a glimpse of my backside in white Calvin Klein's as I changed. I was right. I was NOT a 34. I turned towards the retailer with both hands shoved down the pants. They were way too big.

He nodded his head up and down. "They fit good."

"They do not," I countered.

Susan rescued somebody. "You are not at Versace. This is the smallest pair he has judging from the scant inventory…"

Well, there was that. It was settled. I was a 34. The man smiled. I paid for the pants and left.

We met Vice President John Dramani Mahama in his office in Osu Castle, also known as Fort Christiansborg or "the Castle" which housed the government of Ghana from 1957 to 2013. Bare wires lay in the corners where the floors met the walls. More than 50 percent of the ceiling tiles were missing. The word 'castle" required great imagination.

Making our way through it was much like reaching a plane at the airport in Lagos. There were strategically placed security checkpoints and at each a "contribution" was needed. The metal detectors didn't work because of an electrical shortage. We were practically strip searched, Susan more than the rest of us. Good thing she wore underwear that day.

Finally, in the inner sanctum of Osu Castle, we waited our "turn" seated on bad leather sofas—like the ones in the Oba's palace. Maybe a job awaited me in this country too. Once inside the Vice President's office, our meeting was brief. A photograph was taken with him in front of a framed photo of the VP with

President and Mrs. Obama during their 2009 trip to Ghana. It was the final stop of one of the US President's first international trips.

Susan told him her daughter Ellie went to school with our President's daughters in Chicago when he was still a senator. The VP asked if Ellie was invited to stay with them in the White House. When Susan said "no," we were dismissed.

John Dramani became the Ghanaian President following the death of his predecessor, John Atta Mills, July 24, 2012. Then he was elected to serve a full term in the December election. He is the only Ghana President to not have a second term.

ISTANBUL NOT CONSTANTINOPLE

After being exposed to the totally different culture of Africa, I realized varying cultures ignited my creativity. Observing them provides a more intimate perspective of the world and its diverse lifestyles. I enjoy sharing some of those experiences with my friends and clients. Hoping to give them stories to tell their friends and family about their irreplaceable travels with their designer.

My immensely successful "pool party" in Nice with side trips to St. Paul de Vence and Monte Carlo (where we got kicked out of the casino), made my best friends and clients wanting to know where the next exotic destination was going to be. Egypt was on the top of my list, but with the political upheaval after the revolution against then-President Hosni Mubarak, it was the wrong time. Instead, I chose another ancient land… Istanbul.

Spanning both Europe and Asia, Istanbul's history dates to the Greeks' settlement there, Byzantium. Through centuries, palaces were built, abandoned, demolished, and rebuilt.

Mehmed II, a 23-year-old Ottoman sultan, conquered Istanbul two millenniums after the city was established. Within 10 years of his victory in 1453, four royal palaces were built.

Steven was not able to get away. Unable to travel alone, AJ accompanied me. Even though she is a United Airlines flight attendant, I bought her a business class ticket on American Airlines. Almost 40 years later she and I were still close. She attended every one of my "pool parties" at the Beverly Hills Hotel and in Nice.

After an 11-hour flight, we were greeted at the gate by our personal tour guide extraordinaire, Ayden. He took care of every detail so when AJ told him I needed a candy bar QUICKLY, he made it happen. Our group totaled 17 including John Cusack and his friend, actor Ned Bellamy. They caught up with us after attending a film festival in Kazakhstan.

We stayed in the Ciragan Palace Kempinski Hotel located on the Bosphorus. Modern buildings have been constructed guarding an authentic Ottoman Palace with views of Istanbul's exotic skyline.

The Muslim's call to prayer echoes down every street five times each day starting at sunrise. There are mosques all over the ancient city and the ezan is chanted in unison for three to five minutes. For tourists not knowing what to expect, it is like the near deafening Dolby Surround Sound you experience in a movie theater.

On a sunny but breezy Sunday afternoon we cruised the Bosphorus. The traffic jam on the international aqua highway is like driving on the 405 in Los Angeles. There were breathtaking fortresses, palaces, and mosques on both the European and Asian sides of the city which we toured for days.

Dolmabahçe Palace, built by Sultan Abdülmecid I in 1854, is the largest in Turkey. It covers an area of 461,250 square feet, contains 285 rooms, 46 halls, 6 hammams, 68 toilets and was built at the extravagant cost equivalent to $1.9 billion in today's (2022) dollars. The interiors combining Rococo, Baroque, Neoclassical, and Ottoman elements, with impressive, frescoed ceilings are way over the top. Featuring heated floors, it is the Winter Palace to our hotel's Summer Palace. I marveled at the details and craftmanship.

Topkapi Palace, built in the 15th century, was home to sultans of the Ottoman Empire until the 19th century. Opulent courtyards featuring intricate hand-painted tilework link a labyrinth of sumptuously decorated rooms. A Harem (for the sultan's many concubines), the Second Court with its vast kitchens and the Third Court containing the sultan's private rooms amazed us all. What was achieved half a millennium ago was unbelievable.

The Hagia Sophia Mosque requires tourists to remove their shoes. My foot was wrapped in bandages, so I did not dare take mine off. Gratefully, I was allowed to put disposable hygienic coverings over them to experience what art historians call the 8th wonder of the world. Built in 537 AD this Byzantine architectural marvel was for almost a millennium after its construction, the largest cathedral in all of Christianity. Then, it was converted into a mosque, then a museum, and then again, a mosque. The interior is known for its enormously wide dome seemingly suspended from the sky and beautiful mosaic scenes that cover the walls of this amazing interior.

Everyone was in awe of the history and culture of this mysterious but friendly city. We dined al fresco, partied at different nightclubs and visited an underground Turkish bath dating back to ancient Roman times.

One morning we were treated to a private tour of the actual hotel palace by the general manager. It was adorned with antique candelabras, jardinières, 19th-century carafes, and Baccarat crystal chandeliers and balusters. Proudly he unlocked the doors to the original Islamic inspired bath built in 1872. Its marble floors, walls, ceiling, columns, and articulated half walls were far more detailed than anything I could design or instruct my vendors to produce. We were flabbergasted at the 5,000 square foot Sultan Suite. Host to guests including Elton John, Oprah Winfrey and Princes Caroline, it is one of the largest and most expensive in all of Europe.

That same day, the manager phoned saying he was upgrading me to a duplex in the actual Summer Palace. He sent a few butlers to my room to gather my belongings hoping not to interrupt our plans. Jumping up and down I reacted like a little kid.

No other guests were staying in the majestic palace, so I used not just my suite but the public spaces as my own. On our last night I hosted a farewell dinner party for our group. Drinks and appetizers were served in my apartment. I wanted everyone to enjoy the close-up views of the river and ancient city's illuminated skyline. Dinner was served at a long table in the elegant crystal, marble and gilt lobby. Before desert we stood on the terrace watching fireworks over the Bosphorus illuminating all the domes and turrets.

At one point, John Cusack turned to me and said, "It is so nice to be treated like a normal person…" I knew what he meant.

No paparazzi. No fans hounding him for autographs or photos. Although we were all his fans, we played it down.

I suggested we take a good look around. Admiring the highly crafted workmanship of the Ottoman imperial palace, we were like sultans. "John, normal people don't live like this," He smiled and nodded his head.

When the party was over, I took a long bath in the hand-carved marble tub in my bathroom. It was an exhausting 11 days, although one of my utmost favorite holidays ever, but I needed a vacation from this vacation. A nice hot bath would help me relax. I immersed myself in the warm water. Without thinking I did not wrap my left foot in a plastic garbage bag taping it shut as I had been doing for years. I just climbed in and fell asleep.

Stupid. Stupid. Stupid.

Our plane departed the next morning, and I did not get a vacation from my vacation once I returned to Chicago. Within one month of the exciting voyage, fever and chills returned. My foot was teeming with a variety of bacteria.

Before I knew it, I was back on IV antibiotics. Another PICC line. My home health care nurse started making house calls again. The line became clogged forcing a trip back to the hospital to have it removed and replaced. The doctor who inserted the new one said my veins were badly scared and if I ever needed another line, they would have to put it in a vein in my thigh.

Several days later I received an urgent call from a realtor asking me if I could meet her at Trump Tower RIGHT AWAY. She was working with a client who was going to need my services.

I told her I could not.

She whispered this would be a very important client and I'd be glad I made the effort. It's not that I wasn't interested, I was always interested in a new client, but I felt awful. It was only 10:30 AM, my nurse had come and gone. I was feverish and tired. All I wanted to do was hide in my bed all weekend.

But the realtor already sold her client on the Trump "expert", the designer who had remodeled and designed more condominiums in the building than any other. So, I put on my uniform and hopped into a cab.

When I was introduced to Marjorie Harvey, from Atlanta, I didn't have a clue who her husband was. Maybe a sports team manager? It didn't matter. She was stunning and exquisitely dressed. A real fashionista. That's when I learned the Steve Harvey family was moving to the Windy City because, since Oprah closed shop, we needed a new celebrity talk show host. They were renting an 88th floor condo. With 16- foot ceilings and floor to ceiling windows it was 6,325 square feet. Even with nothing in it the space is magnificent. I was thrilled I did not take a nap.

I showed Marjorie and her real estate brokers a home in the building I created so they could experience the quality of another installation. She hired me on the spot. When the meeting ended, I did not go home to climb into bed. I was too excited. Instead, I walked to my office to send her a follow up e-mail. Time was of the essence. They needed their new home finished by June 1 and it was already Easter.

Despite the short amount of time their home turned out fabulous. We designed the living room around an exquisite suite of upholstered furniture from Donghia, a leading high-style luxury manufacturer. An antique black lacquered Bechstein concert grand piano was centered in the window flanked by two enormous palm trees. The dining room had a raw edge walnut table surrounded by chairs I designed taking inspiration from Marjorie poured into a Tom Ford zipper dress. She wore that dress beautifully. We commissioned an enormous abstract painting, to breathe life into the room and used dramatic modern art everywhere, even in the kids' rooms. The master bedroom suite was elegantly over the top, but I am not one to kiss and tell. It was their private sanctuary not to be shared with anyone but each other. We also designed another, much smaller condo in the building. It was the classroom for Wynton and Lori who were homeschooled.

Once, I passed out in the Harvey residence. Steve was at work, but Marjorie was home with her personal assistant. We were seated in the living room when I rolled off an ottoman and onto the floor. A new design assistant from my office was with me. Julie did not bring the bottle of orange juice, as instructed, and had no idea what to do so she called our headquarters. Maxine told her to get something anything sugary in me. Marjorie ordered a piece of chocolate cake from the hotel. It didn't take too long for me to recover.

Grateful for Steve's success, he and Marjorie founded a non-for-profit organization to help fatherless kids and cultivate the next generation of responsible leaders by providing one-on-one mentoring. Once a year, it hosts an annual Gala fundraiser which John Robert Wiltgen Design supported. Ads in their program, a table to these gorgeous black-tie events chaired by Steve's twin daughters Brandi and Karli, and outrageous auction items. That is how my Steve and I ended up in Capetown, South Africa. I was the winning bidder for a trip that included airfare, a 5,000 square foot penthouse suite in a fabulous hotel with our own private pool and 24-hour butler. Some of my friends and well-traveled clients met us there. Everyone agreed it is one of the most beautiful countries we ever visited.

After 5 years in Chicago, the Harveys packed their bags and moved to Beverly Hills. Steve's a work-a-holic. He hosts his radio show in the early morning (like when it is still dark outside) and then tapes two episodes of his TV show. In-between all that he writes books and screenplays. He said, for the little time he gets to spend outside he prefers to see sunshine every day.

Recently, the Harvey's moved back to Atlanta buying a small, 35,000 square foot home, set on 17 acres. It was built by and for Tyler Perry who is rumored to have spent $40,000,000 on the construction. Marjorie always admired Tyler's home and now it's hers.

OUT OF AFRICA

In October 2012 Susan and I made our 12th visit to Nigeria. I was extremely sick, but as the leaders of the pack, we had to be there. I swore allegiance to my client promising he would not be bothered with any of the details concerning this project. Running a 102-degree fever when we left Chicago made me determined to recover while in flight.

The site meeting was held in a hot, crowded, smelly trailer with no circulation. Twenty people attended. Since the project was being paid for by the State of Lagos, the Department of Works and Infrastructure totaled the largest number of attendants. Members of the engineering firm were present, as was the general contractor, and project design firm, JRWD Nigeria. I had to open a business in Nigeria to work there.

Quite a bit of construction was completed since Susan and I were last there in August. That wasn't necessarily a good thing. The main house was not built according to my plans. There were columns placed where they shouldn't have been. I was livid. Despite the exacting details incorporated into our drawings the local laborers were used to building homes their own way. It was the job of the general contractor to supervise the construction daily. However, the project was too far along for the team to correct the mistakes.

When the meeting ended Susan rushed me back to the hotel. I was burning up. We didn't leave our rooms. I had to get my fever down, so we could travel home.

The entire time we were in Nigeria, Susan kept texting Steven back in Chicago telling him my condition and symptoms. In return he gave her the best medical advice he could given the circumstances. Insisting I sleep with the connecting door to her room open, she checked on me every hour of the night resulting in absolutely no rest for her. Nor the few days that followed.

Having been sick so many times before, I thought I was invincible. But this time I was closer to death than ever. During all the trips to Africa, I hid the problems with my foot, the infections, PICC line and IV antibiotics. None of us told Fola or the Senator or His Excellency. This was different. Susan finally gave in and asked Fola about the best hospital in Lagos. However, no one he knew ever went to a hospital there. Fola's friends and family either went to London or the US when they needed medical attention.

It seemed like forever before we left for the airport. My fever spiked to 104. Susan was afraid they wouldn't let me board the plane. I saved my best-looking shirt and suit for the ride wanting to appear distinguished and healthy. As always, Fola, and his two attendants, escorted us as far as they were allowed in the airport. Giving each of us a big hug, he promised he would see us soon. He cautioned Susan to take good care of me, then ordered me to get well. Standing at the head of the security line, he waited until we cleared the first checkpoint.

Threatened by security to give them money took all my energy. Being frisked at various check points confused those attendants. They never knew what to do about my insulin pump. Asking me to remove it, I told them I could not and offered to show them how it was attached to my ass. Of course, I take it off every time I shower but I was afraid it would mysteriously disappear. Security examined everything in all our bags. Then, there was the required 'hand job' at the gate.

"I've had sex with less contact than this" Susan told a guard. As black as he was the security man blushed. That's why I love her. She's more irreverent than me.

Afraid their VIP lounge was germ-filled we wouldn't sit down without wiping our chairs and table with anti-bacterial wipes. We carried them with us everywhere we went. I called Mommy to tell her we were coming home. I didn't say anything about how awful I felt.

As expected, the Lufthansa gate attendants were not going to let me board. Whispering to each other they finally told us of their concerns I might be contagious, even though I smiled. Susan had to break a few balls to get us on the plane to Frankfurt. Nothing was going to keep me in Nigeria. She told Steven, if necessary, she would check me into a German hospital. Otherwise, our connecting flight was three hours later.

My fever soaked three T-shirts on the plane. Susan threw each one of them away. In Germany, we were met at the gate with a wheelchair which I hated. I didn't want to appear old and feeble but there is no way I would have made it if I had to schlepp me and my bags through customs to the lounge. It was a hike, and I was so dehydrated I was dizzy and confused.

Finally. Steven met us at O'Hare Airport. It was so good to see him. He spoke to Dr. Lee who said he should take me straight to the hospital, but I refused. I fought to go home and sleep in my bed one more time—in case it was the last.

I was admitted two days later and FINALLY, after 29 years of fighting cellulitis and osteomyelitis, I agreed to let the surgeons chop off part of my left leg. Mom says I should say "amputate" but I think "chopping off" sounds stronger!

After preliminary exams, the surgeon said I should go home for a couple weeks to "get things in order."

That was reassuring. At least he didn't use the word "death".

I told him absolutely not. My things were in order. If he didn't amputate my leg right then and there, I would not let them do it two weeks later. They could not give me more time to think about it. When was the next available time in an OR when they could make half my leg disappear?

Three hours later I was being ushered into the operating room. Mom called. Steven, walking by my side, answered my cell phone. No one said anything to her, but she sensed something was wrong and asked if I was in the hospital. I couldn't lie. What if I didn't make it? I confirmed I was headed into surgery. Finally, they were going to take my leg off—well, half of it to be more exact. I told her I didn't want to die. There were still too many things I wanted to do.

She started to cry.

As much as we loved the excitement of it all, Susan, Ray and I never returned to Africa. During one of our trips, we investigated secure two-bedroom apartments to rent so we'd have our own space to hang out in and somewhere to leave our essentials. Less things to travel back and forth with. But a nice place with 10' tall doors and 12' ceilings, security, a water purification system, and generator were the equivalent of $20,000.00 US per month. And most places in Nigeria require a year's rent paid in full, in advance, particularly from ex-pats. So that didn't happen.

During his term as governor of Lagos, my client quietly passed a law providing for the construction of private homes for himself and future retired governors paid in full by the State.

How's that for a golden parachute? Makes you want to take up sky diving.

The commission to design the estate in Lagos was the highpoint of my career. When we were there, we felt like we were in a James Bond film. Kings. Politicians of the highest level. Bodyguards. Private planes. The unknown. When asked if I would do it again, all things considered, I enthusiastically reply, "Absofuckinglutely."

His Excellency's two-acre estate was designed to be suitable for entertaining weighty politicians from around the world. The huge complex which JRWD Nigeria poured its lifeblood into creating is still a work in progress 10 years later. I am told my client and his wife may move in by 2022. (They were originally supposed to move into this home in 2012.)

Considering he once drove a cab in Chicago while attending Chicago State University, things turned out quite well for the Asiwaju of Lagos. He is running for President of Nigeria in the 2023 election, and seen as one of the frontrunners.

RUNNING UP
THAT HILL

Back from surgery, I neglected to hang the do not disturb sign on the door. Around 6:30 am Friday an army of doctors, interns, and nurses marched in to examine my stump.

I hate that word.

I didn't look. I couldn't look. Susan rose from the couch where she'd been napping. She wouldn't leave me in my room alone, not for one minute.

Someone in the medical legion tried to sound optimistic. "It looks good…" Others nodded in agreement.

How can a leg that had just been chopped in half look GOOD?

When the group finished studying me, someone low on the totem pole re-wrapped the remnants of my leg. I was still groggy and tried to drift off to sleep. I didn't want to think about anything.

Three days earlier Susan and I were in Africa. Despite the state of my health, it was glorious. The fiery sun tanned our bodies as the warm heavy breeze wafted in from the Atlantic.

People smiled broadly and laughed their big loud laughs. I was so sick. Near death.

Should I have stayed there and parked myself on a chaise lounge?

What would Steven think of me now with a leg and a half? (Which is nothing like a foot and a half!) That was my main concern.

My client, Ellen Saslow, once told me her dad was never quite himself after his leg was removed. She warned me repeatedly against agreeing to an amputation. Perhaps that is why I fought so hard and for so long. After designing two luxury high-rise condominiums for her and her husband and then building a 12,000 square foot house for them once they started to make children, that family knew almost everything there was to know about me.

Susan went back to the sofa to rest a bit more. She was exhausted.

When nurses helped me from bed for the first time, I was wobbly and unbalanced. According to my electronic smart bed I just lost 12 pounds.

I don't recommend chopping off half your leg as a weight-loss technique. Even if you're desperate.

I left the hospital on Saturday. After 48 hours, there was no point in hanging around. A physical therapist gave me a passing grade in the art of crutch use.

Ray brought me home. He had been in Brazil 48 hours ago when I was in surgery, but as soon as he received the news he immediately returned to Chicago. Mom and Marty greeted us at my new condo. While in the hospital, one of my subcontractors installed grip bars in my bathroom. But I returned to a construction site. My new dream home was strewn with two-by-fours, sheets of drywall, electrical supplies and dust. Cleaning was Mom's original intention, but everything was covered by it. EVERYWHERE.

She removed the plastic tarps protecting my bed and changed the linens. Mom planned to cook, but guess what? No kitchen. It was gutted months ago while I was still living in the Egyptian Temple. I didn't have a kitchen for nine months after leaving the hospital. That's what's great about Lean Cuisine. Dishes and a dishwasher not required.

Even with my experience, hopping around on crutches while trying to get a meal into the microwave was challenging. Removing the hot plastic tray was a circus act.

Jeff brought me an office chair with five casters making life easier. I sped from my bathroom (where there was a full size Sub-Zero frig), across the new bedroom carpeting, down the hallway to the kitchen and then threw the Butternut Squash Ravioli into the microwave. Nuked it for six minutes and voila! Dinner is served.

Staring at the remnants of my left leg was sickening. Unwrapping it before maneuvering into the shower was the worst. My new morning routine started with a walker to get from my bed to the bathroom. Sit my ass down on the cold marble tub deck to unwrap the dressings. Stand on one leg with the aid of the walker and hobble to the shower. Open the frameless shower door with one arm while balancing on the walker with the other. Grab a grip bar in the shower. Let go of the walker. Lift myself over the shower curb. Lower myself into the teak armchair. Sit there for a long time. Half an hour. Sometimes 45-minutes. Occasionally I fell asleep, hot water rushing over my body, before proceeding with the balance of my morning routine. Every day for the rest of my new life. This was new life #3 not counting any of my past lives. When Steven and I headed out for Sunday brunch my crutches enabled me to hobble the equivalent of a full city block. That was the distance from my front door to the building's passenger elevators. The Egyptian Temple was almost adjacent to those elevators. I'm ashamed to admit I wasn't strong enough to make the trek without stopping more than once to catch my breath. But the exercise was great for my biceps!

I repeated the crutching from home to elevator Monday morning when I went to work. I tried to remember to carry everything I needed. Briefcase. Keys. Wallet. Cell phone. Pre-crutches, it usually took two or three attempts out the door and down the hall before I had it all together. I no longer enjoyed that luxury. I didn't have the energy to waste going back and forth.

The workmen involved with my home renovation were amazed at the speed with which I returned to work. For me, staying home was never an option. I didn't want any more than the two days of down time I spent staring at my new self. It was much healthier to be consumed with office problems, those headaches HGTV never reveals were much easier to bear.

Following 13 years of life in my "Egyptian Temple" several floors below, I bought a bright, south facing, three-bedroom space sight unseen. It had a 60-foot-long outdoor terrace. Since childhood I've dabbled with gardening. Planting seeds, watching them sprout, watering them, weeding, studying their continued growth. Training the Morning Glories to climb the fence. Watching the Night Blooming Primroses snap open after dusk. Harvesting green beans, strawberries, and cherry tomatoes. Now I wanted to recreate that experience.

Six large planters on the terrace containing Clump River Birch, which grew to be almost 20 feet tall, anchored smaller containers filled with bright colored annuals. Exquisite furniture created glamorous outdoor dining and living areas. After nurturing my garden the first season, I realized I needed storage space for cushions and garden tools. That meant a shed, but not an ordinary ready-to-wear shed. No. I designed a Georgian-style temple with the door flanked by two Doric columns and a series of moldings. This architectural gem completed my outdoor retreat.

The guest bedroom's wall of Mondrian-like lacquered cabinetry disguised a Murphy bed and storage space. We rarely have house guests, so it became the yoga room. After being home for one week, Eugene, resumed my core strength-building regime. Fortunately, my physical condition did not gross him out as much as it did me. Solar-powered blinds shielded our activity from becoming entertainment for employees in an office building across the street.

My new home needed work inside and out. The kitchen was in the wrong place. It prevented the great room from being great, so it was relocated to the third bedroom. The cabinetry was wrapped in leather custom dyed and embossed in Italy. Raw silk upholstered walls in the master bedroom offered a comfortable spot against which to bang my head after a doctor's appointment or long day at work. I loved the immediate access to the terrace and realized how lucky I was to be living like this. Even though I was physically challenged I was still living the way I wanted to on my own terms. Always have. Always will.

IN CASE OF FIRE KEEP CALM AND PUT YOUR LEG ON

Mom always fretted about me living alone. The current circumstances turned her hair from gray to white and my niece, Savanna, then turned it blonde. Nonetheless, I managed. I am a survivor. And despite the circumstances, I tried my hand at having fun. As the holidays approached, I tied a colored ribbon around the pant leg covering my much shorter one, adding a bow and ornament for a festive touch.

My friends and family were traumatized, but I assured them I felt much better. No more fever, chills, or shaking. I was healthier than I had been in more than a decade. To prove it, I invited a bunch of them over before Christmas to decorate my new terrace.

Regina flew in from Orange County and we went to a wholesale florist to buy red and silver twigs, lights, and a bunch of ornaments to embellish my outdoor garden. A good time was had by all and reminded us that Christmas is a time when you get homesick—even when your home.

When New Year's Eve rolled around, I was glad 2012 was ending despite all the presents I received that luckily, I could regift. It had been another challenging year. But before the year was over, I received one unbelievable gift that I was keeping for myself…

Steven finally decided to move in with me. It was official.

After years of chatting followed by Friday evenings spent mostly at my house, Steven found the courage to meet me at my office on Friday evenings. He was curious to see my workplace and meet those who worked late with me. A lot of them were Latinas with whom he spoke Spanish. He has a great love for Hispanic culture and the Spanish language. He became a regular fixture in my office after hours and was always interested to see the materials and furniture that gave our projects drama. After that, I slowly started including him at charity functions, award banquettes, and dinners with clients. Everyone loved him.

And I was proud he was my boyfriend—manfriend really. It was a huge change of life for him which took time.

Together, we eagerly anticipated the arrival of my first prosthetic. It was a basic, no-frills model because my stump required another six to eight months to sufficiently shrink before the insurance company would approve a more advanced model. The prosthetist measured, designed, fabricated, and fitted model #1. I practiced walking for him while he diligently made adjustments until I was perfectly balanced.

Remarkably, in about an hour I enthusiastically marched out, hailed a taxi, and 7 minutes later strutted into my office. One by one, my staff members let out piercing cries probably heard in

Argentina. Everyone was thrilled for me. Some of the girls even cried. And they all loved the new pair of leopard print Jimmy Choos on my feet. To wear real shoes again. Not orthopedic oxfords. That was mindboggling. I thought I would never be rid of "the boot".

That same day, Daniela Guini—one of my most valued project managers—and I were interviewed by a potential client in Chicago's newest and most opulent residential real estate development. The prosthetist instructed me to wear my new one, that day, for one hour. No longer! But it took about three hours to tour the spacious condominium and listen to the potential client's list of needs and dreams. We got the job. I was thrilled to receive the new project. Our first of five in the building.

I wore the fake leg for at least six hours before Daniela drove me home. The client had no idea. I didn't want to confuse her. Telling us about her prolapsed vagina, at our first meeting thank you very much, she had enough to worry about. I just wanted the assignment. Finally, back in my own construction site, I ripped off the prosthetic and collapsed into my dust covered bed. It had been a long but glorious first day.

Spring arrived the same time as last year and my clients were inquiring about the 2013 Pool Party. I sent a preliminary itinerary to a select group identifying the destination of Lagos. Highlights included a visit to His Excellency's 40,000-square foot estate. While still under construction, the buildings were up and under roof. The pool party would be at the seashore. A day at Lekki Beach where those, so inclined, could be paddled into the Atlantic to catch fresh fish we would bake for lunch with grilled pineapple picked minutes before and dusted with cinnamon. We might see the Oba in his palace. Perhaps have our pictures taken in the throne room with His Royal Highness. Or on the staircase clad in our own newly tailored traditional Nigerian garb.

Those interested were encouraged to quickly confirm enabling me to choose the best, most secure hotel for our group. I would ask Fola to hire security and find the proper transportation to various locations.

No one RSVP'd. Not one person.

While they enjoyed my cocktail party conversation of the Ivory Coast, fear of kidnapping and terrorism nixed their sense of adventure. While that didn't concern me, perhaps a bus filled with Americans, RICH ones at that, may have been too tempting—even for the most honorable protectors. Stories about such kidnappings appear in the BBC headlines frequently. Therefore, I changed the venue to Florence selecting an old Medici palace as our home away from home. Original frescoes and sculpted reliefs fill the Renaissance-era opulence of the palazzo and convention. Almost 20 people signed up for this destination immediately.

Before leaving for Italy, I spent a few days relaxing with Regina and her family in California. Poolside, my youngest nephew, Justin, was intrigued with my prosthetic. I wondered how it looked through the eyes of a 4-year-old.

"Uncle John, why did you have your leg cut off?" Kids ask the darndest questions.

"Because I wanted to lose weight."

"Uh, uh," he disagreed. "I know why. It's because you have a bad disease."

"You are right," I replied. "I have a bad disease."

***

Fifteen of us were standing in awe of Michelangelo's 17-foot David at the Accademia in Florence. Every day we logged at least six miles on foot. I was exhausted at night but so was everyone else.

Our hotel sat amid one of the city's largest private gardens. Eleven acres of ancient, towering trees with seating areas and superb centuries old sculptures. It was a peaceful place to return to after each outstanding day.

By coincidence, author Dan Brown released *Inferno* several months earlier. Much of the story takes place in Florence. Our guide, Claretta, created a tour taking us to many of the sites in Brown's best seller. Boboli Gardens. The attic above the Salone dei Cinquecento in the Palazzo Vecchio. A secret passage which led from Cosimo I Medici's bedroom to the Arno River. And the isolated Vasari corridor connecting the Pitti Palace to the Uffizi Gallery lined with 16th and 17th century works of art.

There were many stairs and no elevators in these centuries' old structures. Some men in our group helped Steven pick me up by the seat of my pants (no joke—although it could have been funny if they ripped) to assist me climb the massive limestone steps to the principal floor of the assorted palaces on our tour. Everyone was astonished at how well I managed, being new to the world of an amputee. But like my clients and friends, I was determined to have a great time.

Ironically, the avowed centerpiece of our trip—the eagerly-awaited pool party—was forced indoors by an all-day rain. The hotel staff scrambled to make a pair of adjoining salons available to us. While we regretted being unable to be poolside in the hotel's remarkable outdoor setting, rain failed to dampen our spirits or curtail our fun.

Before the festive meal, Steven made a heart-felt speech…

"Everyone, can I have your attention please? I would like to make a toast to all of you in the room and, most importantly, to our host, John. Many of you have been to pool parties around the world with us, but not in a room that was once part of a Medici Palace. This is also the first pool party no one has actually gone into the pool, so for that reason, it is special!"

"John has the vision to create trips as amazing as his designs and I want to share just a little bit of what goes on behind the scenes of the man who makes your world beautiful."

"In the middle of the night I see him crawl to the bathroom instead of putting on his prosthetic, because it is safer for him than risking a fall in the darkened room. We all take this simple task for granted. In the morning, he pulls himself up on the vanity and balances on his walker as he puts his contact lens in the right eye—the one he can sort of see out of. Then, I watch him dress in an amazing suit—you all know what I am talking about—paired now with striking shoes and come out of the closet as a modern-day businessman ready to conquer the world. All of this with a blood sugar level that might be a dangerously low or high. He is truly inspiring."

"Someone once said to me it's a shame John never had a son to carry on the Wiltgen name. I gently reminded them while John would have made a great father, he has left the Wiltgen name on three continents and his creative genius will live on long after he is gone. Many of you in this room have allowed him to create exquisite homes for you—most of you more than one. He humbly proclaims his client's homes are only as beautiful as you let them be."

"I thank you for allowing John and his team into the most private spaces of your lives... your homes, where his legacy will live on. So, please let's all raise our glasses to the fresco on the ceiling of this wonderful salon and give thanks to John, to each other, and to God for all we have been blessed with!"

Steven is an awesome public speaker.

The room was silent except for the sniffles of those who could not hold back their tears.

That same crazy month it was finally time for a new, improved prosthetic. It was a lighter model with a smaller circumference for a better appearance. Recommended for activity levels K2–K4 which has nothing to do with kindergarten, I was K-4. Able to exceed basic ambulation skills, I exhibited high impact and energy levels. A shock absorber and swivel ankle enabled me to dance with practice. It was worthy of the six-million-dollar man I have finally become.

LIVING IN
AMERICA

Steven and I planned to stay home July 4 and veg out. That's short for combining some work in the garden with enhancing my tan line (if the sun was out—which it was).

Between work and appointments with my collection of doctors there was never enough time to accomplish everything on our to-do list. However, that morning, John Cusack's girlfriend Jodi O'Keefe, phoned inviting us to visit them at his sister's farm in Michigan. I hemmed and hawed. The rural southwest Michigan country setting is gorgeous, but traffic from the city is murder unless you travel in the middle of the night which is exactly what John and Jodi did.

We arrived mid-day and connected with them in a quaint rural town as they wandered aimlessly through Main Street's vintage stores and art galleries. It reminded me of Mayberry, R.F.D. but Mayberry had only one diner and no art galleries.

Riding a three-wheeled Can Am Spyder motorcycle, John and Jodi led us to the white farmhouse meandering on 100 picturesque acres. We were greeted with warm hugs from an apron-clad Joan joined by her family. Since it was going to be a while before dinner, she suggested John give us a tour of the grounds. We scrambled onto one of his other three-wheel motorcycles tackling a grassy hill, past a 9-foot "chicken" figurine to the barn.

Joan wanted John to transform the barn into a home, so we climbed off the Spyders for a look. It was empty except for a few cars and garden tools. No insulation. The sun shone through the clapboard. The building rose two stories at the center flanked by lofts. Ideas for converting it to livable space flooded my mind. It needed everything. Clearly a challenging project but it could be fun.

Back on wheels we hit a forested path, forged a stream finally reaching a clearing with a Victorian-style screened gazebo containing wicker seating, dry bar, and well-stocked fridge. John tossed me a much-needed Diet Coke. We were parched. The thermometer read 92 degrees in the shade.

There was either a large pond or small lake on the other side of the clearing. Surrounded by a manicured lawn, the water looked pristine as it gently lapped the teak dock. A peaceful setting when no noise spewed from the motorcycles.

We walked the pier. Always by my side Steven guided me. There was no railing, and my balance was far from perfect. I moved with some trepidation. Not sure what damage would be done to it, I feared falling in the water and drenching my metal and rubber leg.

John asked Jodi if she was going in. She said no, something about her makeup. Jodi always looked like a movie star, but I didn't see any make up. John didn't buy it either. He threw her in. His nephews Dylan and Miles followed. John looked at me, "Come on. Let's go in." He looked at Steven, "You too…"

Steven was nursing a beer and shook his head "no" as he walked to land. John looked at me again. I did not want to go in. That would require removing my leg. I didn't want anyone to see my stump. In my brief post-surgery life, I didn't make a habit of revealing it to many. A few family members but even fewer friends. My world is about aesthetics, making homes and gardens beautiful. Making people's lives beautiful. Underneath my layers of designer clothing, I'm a mess. But I was being challenged. And I didn't want John, or the boys, or Jodi to think I was a coward.

"Okay," I nodded uncertainly. "But I have to take my leg off first…"

Thoughts raced through my head as I sat on the pier. Why did I say yes to Jodi? I could be home, gardening in the privacy of our terrace, working on that tan line. I unbuttoned my shirt and shucked off my pants, then rolled the rubber sleeve of my prosthetic down my thigh setting it off to the side. John helped me stand on one leg and hop to the end of the pier. Then he threw me in.

Whoa!

The water was freezing. But the moment I fell in I loved it. The freedom taken from me before I started having sores on the bottom of my feet returned.

Dylan wanted me to swim to the yellow inflatable raft floating in the middle of the water. I wasn't very good, but I was up for the dare. "Let's go…"

At that moment I decided to have Eugene teach me to swim, not float or play in a pool. Maybe I would train hard, so like Regina and Ray, I could also enter the Alcatraz Sharkfest Swim.

I didn't think about how I would climb up the ladder to get back onto the pier but when I reached it, John and Steven yanked me out of the water. I enjoyed sitting in the sun as I dried off before pulling on my leg.

It was time to eat, and I was hungry. Steven made himself useful. Not only is he an expert in the kitchen but he knows his way around the grill. At home I repeatedly told him he should try out for the reality television cooking competition *Hell's Kitchen.*

Afterwards, John engineered a fireworks display equaling that of the City of Chicago which is broke and has limited money for Roman candles, rockets and other pyrotechnics. Earlier in the day he and his two nephews crossed the border into Indiana and bought out one of the fireworks stores there. The trunk of his BMW overflowed with low explosives. Each produced a variety of effects: noise, colored flames, and smoke. Well, there were some duds.

At one point, Dylan and Miles ran down the hill to retrieve the duds so Uncle John could try to ignite them for us. Joan peered into the vast darkness, warning "Hey you guys...that's dangerous." Looking around, she quipped, "come back here... let Grandma get them!"

The boys emerged from the darkness with a handful of fireworks. They smiled as they handed them to John for a grand finale that combined various effects lasting several minutes.

Savoring the aroma of sulfur, desert was served. While the lemon bars spoke to me, I declined. I was trying to be good.

The night did not end there. We all took a shot at "the chicken." To see it, a couple of the cars were driven into the back yard, their headlights directed on the 9-foot tall "bird". It was a sculpture on steroids with a propane tank affixed to its back. Like visiting a carnival, we all took turns shooting at the tank hoping to blow it up. Each time someone fired the rifle the rest of us stepped back.

"At least you have an emergency room nurse here tonight," I volunteered, glancing toward Steven.

"Oh, perfect. So, we have nothing to worry about," Joan was semi-comforted. "Boys get in the house. It's past your bedtime."

The chicken survived the evening and finally it was time for us to leave. Everyone urged us to spend the night, there was plenty of room, but I did not have the nighttime or morning meds I needed. My evening cocktail of 12 pills was already long overdue.

The next day, Joan sent this e-mail…

Just tried to send you video of the chicken being blown up… It happened!!!! Oh, my goodness!

Was so wonderful being in sync with you as I feel it seems to happen so effortlessly!!! How wonderful!!! So nice to meet Steven and talk and laugh and onwards I say!! Onwards!!

Hope you had great time with our family, and I will see if we can get you the explosion… Omg.

Big hugs. Joan.

BABY YOU CAN DRIVE MY CAR

I wasted no time phoning Eugene proposing we ditch weight-lifting and yoga for a while in favor of swimming lessons. I could float on my back, pretend to do the front crawl, and keep myself from drowning but I had no training in proper breathing or swimming distances.

After Regina's back surgery, swimming was prescribed as physical therapy. She swam every day. At some point she decided to keep on going and trained for the swim from Alcatraz Island to San Francisco. We all went to watch her the first time. It was an emotional family reunion. We were so proud when she climbed out of the Pacific Ocean, legs intact. Accompanied by Ray, they did it two more times.

The first time Eugene threw me in the pool I could barely swim half a lap without being totally winded. We didn't know if I should swim with my water leg. I tried, but it was like a floating device and the foot didn't move so it slowed me down. We quickly learned I performed better without the prosthetic, but that required Eugene's help. I took my fake leg off as I sat in a chair pool side. When I was ready, Eugene pushed the chair toward the edge waiting for me to fall in. Then he'd yell at me, sometimes in Russian, about everything I did wrong. Breathe, two, three, four. Watch your right arm. Turn your left arm out more. Don't hit the water so hard with your hands. Don't kick with your leg. Relax. Keep going. Good. That's good. Repeatedly. Two and three times a week.

People in the know said I looked much better. After all the years I spent fighting osteomyelitis and cellulitis, I had way more energy. The infections were gone. So were the hospital visits, home health care nurses and those blasted PICC lines.

***

Without Steven knowing it, I planned an extravaganza to celebrate his 60th birthday. I booked a small resort in Palm Springs reserving every room with our friends and family.

Since the Ritz in Rancho Mirage is one of our favorite spots, I arranged dinner there for the tribe. Earlier the day of, I wanted to go there to review the seating arrangements and last-minute details. There were 18 of us. While driving down highway 111, I experienced a severe low blood sugar reaction that was so bad, I had no sense of my surroundings. I just finished breakfast but must have taken more insulin than needed. Or the food hadn't entered my system to offset the insulin.

Where was my blind friend Chris when I needed him?

Somehow, I pulled the car off the road and parked inside a gated community. How I got past the guard I'll never know. My hands shook violently. I could hardly grasp my cell phone as I tried phoning Steven. He didn't answer. I called a friend I had on speed dial. Same thing. Then, at the point of passing out, I phoned Jeff. His was the only other number stuck in what was left of my brain. It didn't dawn on me that from Chicago there was little he could do. He answered and recognized something terribly wrong. He said he would track down Steven but told me to hang up and dial 911. Which I did. I think. All I could remember was the voice at the other end telling me to stay on the line. They were tracing my location and wanted me to stay put.

Where was I going?

Jeff reached Steven by calling the hotel. When he delivered the news to everyone at the pool, they all jumped into their cars and began searching for me. As he sped down Highway 111, Steven heard an ambulance. Thinking they were going for me, he followed it and found me passed out in our rental car. He rushed toward the paramedics and explained the circumstances. I needed glucose. They were able to give me glucagon, then orange juice. When I came to and began responding they tested my blood sugar again. It had inched its way back up to 35. I needed more. Slowly my glucose turned to normal. The medics wanted to take me to the hospital. Almost in unison, everyone said 'no". They knew I would be fine. Our friends had seen this before.

Steven drove me back to the hotel. From that moment forward I never drove again. Not a rental car. Not my car. Nada. It is too dangerous to others to have me in the driver's seat. Two thousand fifteen was the last time I drove. I miss it. I've always enjoyed driving and the freedom of being able to get in my car at a whim and wander aimlessly through Chicago neighborhoods. Or any city. Steven doesn't enjoy driving but I love it.

That night, in the mountains at the Ritz overlooking the desert valley, I was fine. Steven, still unaware of his birthday celebration, suggested we cancel dinner, but I wouldn't let him. I wanted one night to be about him.

Aunt Bea sat next to Steven and although she cannot see she commented, "this crowd does not look like they drink very much."

To which Steven replied, "Bea. That's because you cannot see. This group is filled with big drinkers. Well, except for John."

"Good," she was so happy. "In that case I will have a Dirty Martini in a water glass with three olives on the side. I don't want them taking up any space in my glass."

Tears flowed freely as each guest spoke about how Steven impacted their lives. Even after Miss Hollywood presented him with a gift wrapped like artwork, he didn't comprehend the dinner was in his honor, until the cake was brought out and we sang to him.

I LOOK
TO YOU

It was the first Thursday of February 2017. I met Eugene at the Intercontinental Hotel where he continued to teach me how to swim in their junior Olympic pool. The blue fish scale-patterned stained-glass windows, traditional ceiling, stone columns, pilasters and Neptune themed fountain make me imagine I'm swimming in the Alhambra. Johnny Weissmuller, winner of five Olympic gold medals and star of 12 Tarzan movies trained there.

Ever since John Cusack threw me off the pier into the cold lake on his sister's farm, I decided to learn to swim. When Eugene was a kid, he used to be on a Russian swim team in Moscow, so he was the perfect coach.

When we were kids, Mom was a Wichi Wachee Mermaid at the local YMCA and taught us to hold our breath, dive, and float on our backs. As a child, I jumped from the high diving board at our park district's pool. At Grandpa's house in Tomahawk, he pulled us on a raft behind his speed boat. As we went 'round and 'round in small circles, the waves got gigantic. We would crash through them trying to hold on. I always loved that time in the water.

Even if I got a leech or blood sucker on the bottom of my foot.

Breathing in the water was the hardest part for me. I never learned how to do that correctly. For months I paddled back and forth (two laps) with my head always above water. I would stop, clean my goggles, catch my breath, talk and then swim two more laps. After lots of practice, I finally got my breathing right. I was swimming more laps without stopping and it felt great. That night in February I swam my personal best; six sets of 10 laps in the least amount of time.

When we finished Eugene pulled me out of the pool and put me in a chair so I could pull on my leg. I had a bit of a cough and he recommended I sit in the sauna to burn it out. Sitting on the warm teak bench, I began coughing mercilessly. Thankfully, I was the only one in there. The veteran who ran the health club heard me from outside the locker room and brought me two cups of cold water.

"You alright?" he asked.

"Yeah, I'm fine. Thank you."

After I finished, I waited on a cold, rainy, Michigan Avenue for Steven to pick me up. He came for me after every swim. On the way home we talked about how well I was doing. He congratulated me knowing how important this was to me.

Friday, after work, I went straight home. I did not meet Steven and our friends at a bar we frequented to celebrate the end of the week. I did not feel good. I was coughing non-stop and needed rest. After drinking a cup of hot tea I climbed into bed propping myself up with multiple pillows hoping that would make it easier for me to breathe through the night.

Saturday, I sat in one of the swivel chairs in our living room all day. I didn't move. I didn't swivel. I drank more tea and watched the Netflix series *Versailles*. As much as I was enjoying it (I wanted to live there), I kept fading in and out of the show, blaming it on the comfort of the chair.

Sunday, ditto. Except I finished *Versailles'* first season and hoped they would produce more. Steven made some Jewish penicillin commonly known as chicken soup. But it didn't help. Probably because he isn't Jewish.

It was late and I had to shake this cough. Tuesday I was supposed to fly to Dallas to meet with clients and help them select "red carpet appropriate" jewelry to don with a gold sequin Tom Ford dress she was wearing to the Elton John Academy Awards Afterparty. After taking all my drugs I climbed into bed, propped up with the same stack of pillows I used the night before, and coughed and coughed and coughed…

Steven had just taken the only pill that helps him sleep. In about five minutes he would be out, despite my hacking.

"I think you should go to the hospital…" he said.

"Okay," I acquiesced. I really couldn't breathe.

He called for an ambulance.

After a quick assessment that determined my oxygen saturation was in the low 80 percent range (normal is in the high 90's), the paramedics strapped me to the gurney, wheeled me down the corridor complaining the whole time it is a block long and loaded me into their ambulance. After seeing me safely inside and providing the paramedics the necessary details about my health, Steven was too drowsy from his medication to accompany me. He felt awful, but I assured him I would be fine. The paramedics tried to make me comfortable before announcing I would not be able to go to the hospital where all my doctors practice. It was on "bypass". There were no beds available. Well, except in the morgue.

Instead, they rushed me to another university medical center. That began a 21-day, near-death stay I wouldn't wish on anyone.

When Steven arrived Monday morning, I was in a stark white, isolated ICU room. Everyone entering had to wear disposable gowns, masks, and gloves. I felt better. Tuesday, I sat in the chair, ate the hospital food, and conversed much more comfortably than the previous day. If my condition improved, we expected me to be discharged by Friday or Saturday. That belief was short-lived.

After two days without IV fluids Steven finally convinced the doctors they were damaging my kidney. Having just celebrated my 30-year transplant anniversary my lab values showed I could be heading into renal failure. Dehydration is extremely dangerous to anyone, but even more so to a kidney transplant patient. As soon as I received a couple bags of IV saline, my kidney functions improved.

On day three my temperature began to rise, and my oxygen levels plummeted. I coughed so hard and so often I should have died of exhaustion. My oxygen supply was increased to the max to keep my levels as close to normal as possible. I was on high flow oxygen and getting breathing treatments every four hours. Coughing up an endless amount of mucus, it was getting thicker.

Every day an entire medical lineup converged outside my room to discuss me and my case. Pharmacists, nutritionists, respiratory therapists, physical therapists, nurses, interns, residents, attending physician's, fellows etc. reviewed my progress or lack thereof. The lab results showed I had Respiratory Syncytial Virus (RSV) an illness that mostly affects children or the elderly. Antibiotics are ineffective against viral illnesses so the hospitalists could do little besides give me more fluids, Tylenol for the 103-degree fever, and rest.

Steven attended every Medical Rounds Meeting giving valuable information often overlooked by those who saw me for minutes a day. His medical background enabled him to ask relevant questions, share his own assessment, and remind them of tests and treatments they were going to order but did not. If he had not been there as my advocate, I would not be writing this. Every patient needs a family member or friend who can listen, think, and be their voice when they are hospitalized.

In that first week, I had three chest X-rays. One morning a doctor came into my room asking if I had seen them. I shook my head "no". It hurt too much to talk. He turned the computer screen toward my bed, pointing at the first one taken when I was admitted. Then he showed me the third. It was completely white which, he explained, is terrible. My infection was way worse.

A CT scan was ordered. The doctors needed to see the minutiae the scan offers. I was afraid I would not be able to lie flat and stay still. I lived in the upright position day and night coughing and spitting as I tried to get the phlegm out of my lungs.

I was transported, in my bed, to the location of the CT scanner. Steven came with, he wouldn't let me out of his sight.

The technician greeted us and helped move me to the table for the scan. And in that moment, I knew…

"Where are you from?" I inquired, even though it hurt me to speak.

"I am from Nigeria," he replied proudly.

"Lagos?"

"Yes. How did you know?" I had his attention.

"I have been there many times." He and his female assistant, both from Lagos, were so happy and tremendously kind. Steven told them about my work there, my visits to see the Oba (their eyebrows went way up into their foreheads,) and our recent trip to beautiful South Africa. They were thrilled to hear someone, particularly a white someone, say something nice about Africa, Nigeria and its people. That experience was the most pleasant part of my stay.

After a week, I showed no improvement. It was decided by the "team" to examine my lungs with a lighted scope, called a Bronchoscopy. I kept saying I didn't want them to, but Steven swore it necessary. I trusted him more than anyone. The procedure was done bedside.

One of the doctors inserted giant Q-tips in my extremely tender nose to apply a numbing medication. I also received a dose of something I swished in my mouth that tasted like poison to numb more of me. Then, through my IV a liquid drug was supposed to induce a twilight sleep. However, the pain from them shoving the Bronchoscope through my nose and into my lungs was so bad, Jeff, who waited in the hallway outside my room, heard my ear-piercing screaming.

I've had twilight sleep before, and this wasn't it.

When they inserted the long tube up my nose and down my throat (raw from coughing for days) I gagged and choked and prayed I would die. Steven stayed by my side the entire time.

The next day was worse. The benefit of the Bronchoscopy came with a side effect of increasing the inflammation in my lungs. My temperature soared. We were told my lungs were completely coated with a fungus, Thrush. The mucus showed Hemophilus Influenza was also there. This can cause middle ear infections, sinusitis, and more serious infections including meningitis. Most strains of this live in their host without causing any problems, however, when other active viral infections create an opportunity, they attack the human body. To make matters worse, the mucus also revealed I had Coronavirus (not to be confused with COVID 19 but bad enough) and Staph Aureus in my blood.

How did I get all these infections at the same time?

In 2017 many people were hit hard by the flu. Roughly 40,000 people in the U.S. die from it each year. When my system was attacked by one infection, other viruses and bacteria took over my weakened immune system. Two of my doctors were flabbergasted. They never saw this severe a case of pneumonias in someone STILL LIVING.

It was time to ask God for help. Steven went to the hospital chapel two and three times daily. My dire situation was that dire.

Finally, antibiotics and an anti-fungal medication were ordered to reduce the severity of the symptoms preventing my recovery. The deadly combination of infections made me weaker, and I wasn't eating.

Struggling to reduce the inflammation and tightness in my lungs one of the doctors quadrupled my normal dose of Prednisone. It is a steroid. And the larger dose caused me to feel like I was tripping on some nasty psychedelic drug. A million fragmented images of my life flashed through my brain non-stop. I wasn't sleeping so I couldn't shut it off. Distorted, twisted technicolor images ran through my head. It was awful. The increased dosage caused me to retain fluids, so they prescribed IV Lasix, a potent diuretic. That made me pee a lot more often which takes a lot of oxygen.

Who knew?

The nurses had to crank up the oxygen just so I could take a leak. In fact, they had to crank up the oxygen to eat, drink, talk, put on a clean T-shirt, and then take it off.

Later the second week, the infectious disease team finally decided to try an anti-viral drug Steven asked about a week earlier. As my condition deteriorated the doctors were desperate and finally listened to him. For five days I took Ribavirin, a medication used to treat RSV. It can cause anemia increasing heart problems, sometimes resulting in a heart attack. The doctors stopped my other heart medications assuring me the risk of a heart attack was less than the chance of me dying from the multiple lung infections.

At this point, Steven was terrified I would not make it. I told him I did not have the energy to keep fighting and he should let me go. He started to weep.

I thought he might be a lot better off without me and all my health bullshit.

"Just hold on" he pleaded.

On three different occasions he phoned Ray and Susan, requesting they come to the hospital quickly. He thought I was leaving—and I don't mean for a trip around the world.

As my oxygen level became dangerously low, I said to him "I want to be able to tell everyone goodbye". Someone said Regina was on her way from California and I thought, "I must really be going. I hope First Class".

And then the most astonishing moment of my life occurred.

I was not conscious. Steven had been praying constantly. All our family and friends were praying their hearts out. It was early morning. Sorrowfully Steven believed my time had come. He looked at me and then the ottoman next to my bed. Sitting there he saw Jesus. My eyes were closed, and Jesus was holding my hand in His. He was ministering to me. Soothing my aching body.

I did not know He came to visit.

Later that day and into the night, every time Steven laid his hand on my chest it was like being touched by God. I was calm and at peace. And my condition improved. I was still coughing and spitting up mucus, but everything seemed easier.

Was it the prayers of so many? Had they been heard? How many hands has Jesus held? How many bodies have been healed by his loving touch?

My supplemental oxygen requirements were minimized enabling me to leave the ICU. After 16 days in isolation, I was transferred to a general medical floor.

As my appetite increased and my ability to get up and move around eased, I finally believed I was going home. Therapeutic oxygen was prescribed, and I was discharged on a simple nasal cannula. On a frigid Saturday evening, three weeks after I entered Rush Presbyterian St. Luke's Medical Center, Steven pulled our car up to the front door of the hospital and with Ray's help, brought me home.

While still confined to the ICU, Steven and I discussed my future, meaning the future of John Robert Wiltgen Design. For 40 years JRWD had not only been my career, but my life. Was it time to retire? I have been blessed with clients who allowed me to create the most extraordinary homes for them, many were award winning. From one coast to another. Mexico. Canada. Even Africa.

Did I think it was time to move on?

Although it broke my heart, the answer was a definite "yes". There were so many other things I still wanted to do.

I'M
STILL HERE

S ince retiring at 57 I am busier than ever…

Steven and I got married. One Sunday, after she came home from church, he asked Mom, a devout Catholic, if it was all right with her. She started to cry. That's what mothers do. I am lucky Mom got over the whole gay thing years ago because her tears were tears of joy. She waited all these years to see her oldest child married. FINALLY! But I know she wondered: was she the mother of the bride or the mother of the groom and did she have to pay for anything?

How about a new Tom Ford tuxedo? Yes, I don't think I told you, but in my old age I have moved on to Tom Ford.

Getting married, especially the first time around, is a big deal. For everyone. It's an even bigger deal if you are two men or two women. In my 59 years on this planet, I had only been to two gay weddings, and one didn't include a ceremony.

My stepsister married her girlfriend in Illinois, way before it was legalized and before she had gastric bi-pass surgery, lost a lot of weight, and then decided to try being straight. That worked for her because she met and married an attorney and conceived a child with him the old-fashioned way. Her former wife has been her son's live-in nanny for 10 years now. I cannot tell you anything more about *that* because this is all I know.

My friend, Willy (from the paint store and disco days) and his partner were married before a judge in Iowa, where gay marriage was legal. They then hosted a celebration of their union back home in Michigan with their nearest and dearest. Designed to be a garden party at their beautiful manse on Lake Michigan of course it rained, a torrential downpour.

These are my experiences with gay weddings.

Regina and I scoured every venue in Chicago for a place to host this celebration, but after days of looking Steven and I ultimately decided to get married in Palm Springs. We did not want the get-together to be over in 6 hours. Instead, we preferred to spend as much time as possible with our family and closest friends.

Aunt Bea, who was 94 at the time, would be able to attend with her boyfriend of 7 years Dr. Joe. That meant the world to us.

Mom and Marty hosted our rehearsal dinner at the steak house in the casino. After dinner on a private terrace, we went indoors to try our luck against the house. I mentored Steven's son and daughter at one of the Blackjack tables. Some of the other youngsters were enamored with the Roulette Wheel from which we heard lots of screaming mixed with cheering.

When it was time to walk back to our hotel there was an unexpected and heavy rainfall. Water was leaking through the recessed lights over the slot machines. I hoped it wasn't that black cloud syndrome returning after so many years of absence.

The service and festivities were held in the Palm Springs Museum of Art. Art played an important role in the homes I created making the museum the most appropriate destination. I provided our DJ a specific list of music to play, and he made a CD for each of our guests. My niece's boyfriend was the officiant which meant two Catholic men were married by the most adorable Jew.

Amid the cocktail hour Regina gently nudged people aside creating an aisle of sorts and the song we selected, *This Is the Moment,* quieted our group. Mother and Steven's daughter, Jenna, gave us away. The two of them wore beautiful white gowns. (Someone had to wear white.) Mom looked like old Hollywood and Jenna, a younger newer star. It was black tie optional giving us an excuse to play dress-up once again. Only, now I no longer needed Mom's eyebrow pencil. I brought my collection of Versace ties with us thinking it would be great if all the men wore one.

We had one long dining table, so everyone sat together. The table was teeming with candelabra, varying in height, that held hundreds of candles. Ray acted as the emcee and gave everyone an opportunity to say something. There were so many stories and tears of joy.

Regina told everyone how frightened she was to accept the assignment of wedding planner knowing how particular I was when it came to design. And how much she loved Steven.

My niece remarked not everyone is fortunate enough to have an uncle buy them a pair of black leather Versace jeans when they are 8 years old. She reminisced about how I would dress her and my other nieces in fabulous designer outfits complete with stockings, shoes, and a handbag. And she finished with how much she loved Steven.

It was unanimous. *Everyone loves Steven.* It should be a TV show.

Those five days were, by far, the happiest of our lives.

As soon as we got home, I became very ill. Of course. Who would expect less of me? Appendicitis. My appendix ruptured in the hospital. At first the doctors thought my kidney was rejecting. For 36 hours, infection (peritonitis) spread throughout my abdomen before they finally decided what was wrong with me. A ruptured appendix can kill you and for that reason Steven did not expect me to survive. Again. But by now, you know, I am a walking miracle.

For real!

Steven retired. We didn't know if I used up the miracles I'd received. We spent months relaxing in the desert cultivating new friendships we will cherish forever. Aside from Palm Springs, one of our trips was to Barcelona. Dan Brown wrote another book, *Origin*, inspiring a portion of yet another journey. The unfinished Antonio Gaudi Roman Catholic Basilica Sagrada Familia looks like it came out of the old tv series *Flash Gordon*. The attic of the private residential building, Casa Mila, also a Gaudi structure, is a work of art. And just like in the book we visited the 11th century Abbey of Montserrat by cable car.

Brown should open a travel agency. The destinations in his books are spectacular!

Even though everyone we encountered spoke English, Steven was able to use his perfecto Espanol. Of course, the locals spoke Catalonian, but they were impressed with his Spanish and replied with it to him.

From Barcelona we boarded the brand-new Symphony of the Seas, an enormous cruise ship built for 6,600 passengers with a crew of over 3,000. We were traveling on its third week at sea. I felt confident I would not have to worry about flus or viruses that germinate on so many of the older ships.

Selfishly, I planned private day tours for our group only. There were specific places I wanted to see that were not on the boat's excursions. My sister Cindy and her new husband, Tom, both who had never been out of the country, traveled with us. It was heartwarming to watch Cindy's eyes continually pop out of her head like ping pong balls. In Cinque Terre she climbed to the very top of an 800-year-old castle. In Rome she and Tom fought the crowds to throw money into Trevi Fountain. In Napoli they were amazed by the historian who led us down the streets of Herculaneum, an ancient city destroyed when Mount Vesuvius erupted.

We returned home and shortly thereafter the WHOLE world changed. It was like Mount Vesuvius erupted again, only all over the globe.

In December 2019 Dr. Li Wenliang, an opthamologist in a hospital in Wuhan, tried to inform others about the erupting virus. Without delay the police accused him of spreading false information and ordered him to stop. Continuing to work, he caught the virus from a patient and died. China did not share this information immediately with the rest of the world. Thirty days later, on January 20, they finally revealed the outbreak of the newest Coronavirus known as COVID 19.

On January 21 the first case of COVID was discovered in the United States. The following day President Trump told the world "…we have it under control. It's going to be just fine."

Soon afterward, the Chinese government closed Wuhan. That is when it made its first impression on our lives. We were still renovating our newest home and some of the products were coming from there. One of our subcontractors was stuck in Wuhan and no one knew when he would return to the States and his family. That made us nervous.

The virus was spreading. Our Commerce Secretary, Wilbur Ross, attempted to put a positive spin on the state of affairs declaring the Coronavirus would help accelerate the return of manufacturing jobs to North America.

President Trump confirmed this by adding "We think it's going to have a very good ending for it. So that I can assure you…"

Meanwhile, the World Health Organization declared a global health emergency warning that people over 60 years old and those with underlying medical conditions (such as diabetes, cardiovascular disease, chronic respiratory disease, HIV, organ transplants and cancer) are at a higher risk for catching the disease and dying.

That included ME.

The extreme illness I endured in 2017 damaged and scarred my lung tissue making it harder for my lungs to work properly when there's nothing wrong with me. The walls of the tubes enabling air in and out of my lungs were also thickened making breathing more difficult. And maybe I have sarcoidosis but since we don't know for sure I'm not going to dwell on that.

Steven and I had serious conversations about this deadly disease. He was glued to the TV as he tried to make sense out of the varying theories and reports coming from our President, the National Institute of Health, the Center for Disease Control, the National Institute of Allergy and Infectious Diseases, the World Health Organization and every doctor, professor, and pharmacologist from around the globe who had an opinion.

When the New York Times revealed the National Security Council's biodefense experts looking into how to quarantine a city the size of CHICAGO we quarantined ourselves. It was hardly a thing yet. None of the States had considered such extreme actions but starting the third week of February, I was confined to the primary bedroom suite. Steven lived in the rest of our condo since he prepares our meals and took care of the rest of life's must do's. He shopped for our groceries, picked up prescriptions but did not visit any family or friends in our home or anywhere else. We detached ourselves for the duration. I could not risk exposure to the deadly COVID 19 virus.

I needed to exercise daily to stay in shape and compensate for all the food Steven was serving. Unfortunately, we did not raise the ceiling in the primary bedroom during our renovation otherwise, I could have used the bed as a trampoline. On our 75″ TV I turned on YouTube and watched old disco music videos trying to dance along. Love the music and the dance moves even though some of them were hard to perfect on carpeting with my prosthetic.

Dance. Watch everything on Netflix. Eat and Facetime. That was my life and for the most part I was OKAY with it. I was NOT going to get this, and our President promised, "…it's going to work out fine."

After several weeks of isolation, I started coughing. Steven and I both felt it was Bronchitis. In the past six months I had been diagnosed with it twice. An inhaler and antibiotics were prescribed both times which provided the remedy. I had a very low-grade, almost non-existent fever of 99 - 99.2 but my oxygen level was normal.

I drank a lot of tea, sipped homemade chicken soup for lunch and dinner and stayed locked up in the primary bedroom. Despite these efforts the cough did not go away.

With all the time and precautions, we took I did not want to go to my doctor's office and risk exposure to COVID 19. I was shocked to learn Dr. Lee's office was open. So many doctors closed their facilities to hold virtual appointments. However, it was inevitable. I had to go. Dr. Lee could not get blood from a virtual meeting.

Steven went to our storage room to find my wheelchair. Before leaving he disinfected every inch of it. Then we each put on rubber gloves and a mask. Once there, I sat in it instead of one of the upholstered chairs in the waiting room sat in by other patients.

Fortunately, the doctors' offices were totally empty minus the nurses and doctors. Dr. Lee examined me immediately believing my symptoms to be Bronchitis. Her office did not have the test for the Coronavirus. I was surprised because on March 6 President Trump announced, "anybody that wants a test can get a test."

The doctor prescribed two antibiotics and another inhaler. This one had steroids in it which could cause Thrush in my mouth, so I was instructed to brush my teeth and gargle immediately after every use.

I was relieved this was another case of Bronchitis, but the prescriptions did not improve my cough. Instead, it worsened.

No longer having the energy to get up and disco dance or dream about the trampoline it kept getting harder to breathe. On several occasions Steven asked if I wanted to go to the hospital.

My answer was always NO. I was so afraid. Afraid #1 the hospital was on lockdown so Steven would not be able to stay with me nor could he visit. Afraid #2 I would be put on a gurney and left in one of the alleged crowded hallways of the hospital. And, afraid #3 if I did not have COVID 19 I would be exposed to it there, get it, and die. I wasn't ready to die, and didn't think They weren't ready for me up there yet.

When I had the chills and it became harder than ever to breathe, I conceded. Those were my symptoms. No fever, headache, muscle pain, or sore throat so I prayed it was a bad case of Bronchitis. Or pneumonia. Either one would be better than COVID. The hospital would figure out the problem.

It was an unusually nice day, so Steven pushed me in the wheelchair to the emergency room. We live two blocks away from the emergenncy room and he felt we'd be there faster than waiting for the paramedics.

At the automated glass doors, we were greeted by a hospital employee who took hold of my wheelchair and told Steven he could not enter. It was frightening and heartbreaking for both of us. What if I died and we never saw each other again? Steven stood outside and cried.

Except for the staff, who were all in disposable gowns, gloves and masks, the emergency room was empty. It was just me and them. After a nurse took my vitals someone else pushed me down a long empty corridor into a glass enclosed examination room. I was told to put on one of those depressing hospital gowns before being interviewed by several different doctors, each at different times, about my history and current symptoms. I repeatedly told each of them I had a bad case of Bronchitis. Before long I was transported to an isolated room on a designated Coronavirus floor.

That was shocking. Why was I there? I would, for sure, become infected with the deadly virus. Was this the end?

A nurse took blood from both arms and then hooked me up to an IV. The hospital did have the COVID test which involved, once again, sticking huge Q-tips way up my nose. Who thinks these things up?

By the end of the day the test came back. Positive. I had COVID 19.

How could that be when I quarantined in my master bedroom for so long?

Every day the nurse assigned to my care phoned me before coming to my room during mealtimes and several obnoxious hours when I should have been sleeping. What else might I need before they brought my food, took my vitals and withdrew blood - all at the same visit? There was no going in and out of COVID rooms. To hopefully prevent the spread of the disease to the brave staff, their gowns, masks and gloves were discarded every time they'd leave. Doctors rarely came to visit me. Instead, they called to discuss my most recent lab results and ask how I felt. Several times, one recommended I move to ICU where they would intubate me. I said there was no fucking way anyone was going to intubate me and to make sure, I was not going to ICU. Steven's 30 years of hospital experience taught him long-term high-pressure ventilation combined with the Covid-19 was deadly. No matter what, he was completely against me being put on a ventilator.

As bad as things were, I preferred my room without a view and, more importantly, the en-suite bathroom. It wasn't aesthetically like any of ours at home but at least it was accessible. In ICU I was informed they would not let me out of bed to use the facilities. That just didn't work for me. There was no way I was going to take a dump in a bedpan with someone watching!

To stay alive, I Facetimed Steven twenty times a day and sometimes in the middle of the night. He helped reduce the overwhelming fits of anxiety I experienced. No matter what pill they gave me I didn't sleep so I watched reruns of *Law-and-Order SVU* in the middle of the night.

When I was first admitted, I watched the news, but the constant references to the numbers of people dying and the overcrowding in hospitals did more damage to my psyche than having the virus. Imagine being alone in a semi-sterile room with COVID. The media's constant and relentless doomsday reports did not give me one bit of hope for recovery. What they did was scare the shit out of me and everyone who loved me. Dr. Fauci predicted 100 million people would die.

Mindless TV allowed me to escape this grim reality. By the time I was discharged from the hospital, Mariska Hargitay, the female star who played officer Benson, worked her way up to captain just as I was going home.

Steven believes positive energy and prayer help us improve physically and mentally. He organized a prayer group of about 40 people who texted each other at 11 am and 6 pm every day for 5 weeks. Faithful and true they showed up twice a day, every day, to keep our hope alive.

The most horrific part of COVID 19 is the separation from family and friends. Being sick and hospitalized brings anxiety under normal conditions. The fear of dying in the hospital, alone, impacted me tremendously as well as those who love me. The shattering heartbreak of maybe being lucky enough to say goodbye over the phone was inexpressible. For those whose lives end this way my heart bleeds.

At the height of my illness Steven reached out to our friend who is an undertaker. Since Covid-19 even death has taken on a new meaning. Funerals were limited to 10 people, so who do you ask to attend? The body could not be viewed. Family members like mine may have last physically seen their loved ones when they left them in an emergency room. Steven wanted to be sure the last person who touched my body was someone who cared about me as a person and would be kind and loving. Our friend Brad was a godsend helping Steven develop the next steps if necessary. Steven was comforted knowing if I died, I would be treated with love and respect. These situations were never considered before Covid-19. Our world has certainly changed. Fortunately, their plan never had to be carried out.

I spent 15 nightmarish nights in the hospital where I received great care. Though circumstances like this bring devastation they also bring hope and renewed faith in the goodness of mankind. So many heroes stepped up to the plate way before there was even hope for a vaccine.

Everyone who know me, knows I am a fighter. I have spent my entire life fighting. Fighting to succeed while fighting to survive. Since I was a kid, I always dreamt BIG while fighting not to let negativity complicate my life.

After Steven, John Robert Wiltgen Design is still my greatest passion. With an incredible client base that included celebrities and heads of foreign states, I obsessed over making their worlds beautiful, wherever that world may have been. Fortunately, I am still in contact with many of my clients who have become good friends. Recently, Steven and I had a JRWD reunion with people who worked with me in my office. It was our first real party in our new home. COVID kept us from interacting with people in big groups for an inordinate length of time.

I keep in touch with most of the characters mentioned in my story. I phone my Mom and Aunt Bea almost every day. I talk to my brother and sisters several times a week. Sue, the one who worked with me when I couldn't see, calls me in the morning on her way to her Phoenix office. The other Susan who traveled to Africa with me sends me text messages while waiting in an airport as she travels around the world for work. Happily, I am still in touch with Jeff and we speak often. Steven and I see Daniela, my brilliant assistant for the last 7 years (when I was most sick) and her husband Petr. They are like family to us. Bill divorced Leslie, his second wife. Steven and I just met his next one. She's lovely too. Jimmy calls several times a month no matter which home he's in. Lara lives in Switzerland and recently finished building a magnificent home Steven and I want to visit as soon as COVID restrictions have been lifted. Miss Hollywood and her partner, Robert, come to Palm Springs to visit Steven and me. My good friend Gertrude departed this world. I miss her so but am in touch with her daughter, Karen. I don't hear from Leana or Rhonda but still speak with Jill and A.J.

I saw my life pass before me more times than a cat's lives. There are still things I want to check off my bucket list. Malta. I am dying to go to Malta. They have ruins as old as the pyramids. A walled city, Mdina, where 12th and 13th generation descendants of the Knights of Malta still live in their family's original palaces. I would love to stay in the new petit hotel that opened inside Versailles. At night-time guests are given private tours of the palace after the crowds have left. And I want to go back to Rome and take a private tour of the Vatican before the mad rush and long lines. For that I would get up early in the morning. I would also like to visit the Vatican gardens. Steven and I would love to take a train ride through the Rocky Mountains and end up in Seattle to see his brothers. These are just four things at the very top of our bucket list. We have so many more items.

Hoping to open an exquisite door to a new life, if ever I should tell my story, it is now. So many miracles. There is no other way to explain it.

I want to become an advocate for people from all walks of life who are dealing with similar problems. Through the power of the written word as well as public appearances, I want people to know that with a chronic disabling disease so many things are possible if you are not afraid to dream.

Hopefully, I have inspired anyone who has ever wondered if the next experience is worth fighting for, particularly if you deal with illness every day of your life. To those who are worried over, prayed for, and cried about since they were young, I'm still here to tell you YES, the battle is worth it!

Maya Angelou wrote, "Life is not measured by the number of breaths we take, but by the moments that take your breath away."

I have had my breath taken away so many times because I decided, at a young age, to do just that! I grasp every day with an "I can do anything" attitude. I encourage everyone to do the same.

...to be continued...

www.ingramcontent.com/pod-product-compliance
Lightning Source LLC
Chambersburg PA
CBHW060853120626
46553CB00001B/72